Praise for *Sorry About Your Diagnosis . . . You're Fired!*

"An inspiring, authentic story of resiliency through life's biggest heartbreaks. And, most importantly, a love letter to all the special people in her life—her angels." —**Sam Norpel, Chief Digital Officer, JuvLife, Juvenescence; Alumni Board Member, Women in Retail Leadership**

"Cindy's courage and vulnerability reminds us how our family and friends can provide love, strength, and support. And take each day as it comes, focusing on learning and the possibilities." —**Linh Calhoun, Chief Marketing Officer, Replacements, LTD., Mentee**

"Very few people in today's world speak with the clarity and calm that Cindy brings to hearing and heeding her true inner voice. Each page showers the reader with Cindy's light, peace, and strength (her tough cookieness); a gift from Cindy to us all!" —**Cristina Ceresoli, VP Growth Marketing, Chico's FAS**

"Cindy conveys her story of resilience and positivity with warmth and honesty. She SHINEs through any challenge she faces, encouraging us all to follow her lead and "get on it!" —**Susan Landay, President, Trainers Warehouse**

"Cindy lays bare the travails of real life. Sharing her journey through the weaving path of cancer, she brings one along with her truthful voice. Her story is one of resilience and celebrates the triumph of faith, patience, and gratitude." —**Margot Murphy Moore, Former Chief Strategy Officer/CEO of Hyland's**

"A breathtaking memoir from a courageous woman who, faced with sudden adversity, embraced her circle of love and power, doubled down on her resiliency, and shined." —**Stefanie Jandl, Independent Scholar and Friend**

"In a time when technology and the pandemic have redefined true human connection, Cindy's book illustrates the power of our network. Key to overcoming challenges, our personal connections give us strength and hope, allowing gratitude to lead the way as a seemingly more powerful antidote than medicine." —**Laura Hnatow, Vice President, Marketing and Ecommerce for Sea Bags**

"Cindy is an empathetic, thoughtful, and highly poised leader, mentor, and friend. Her journey is an inspiration."—**Annie Selke, CEO of The Annie Selke Companies**

Published by Black Box Publishing

For more information, contact: info@paulablack.com

ISBN - 978-0-9768285-8-7 (paperback)

ISBN - 978-0-9768285-9-4 (ebook)

Design by: Patrizia Sceppa, Inc.

Printed in the United States of America

Sorry About Your Diagnosis . . . You're Fired!

A story of courage, tenacity, love, and fragility

Cindy Marshall

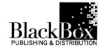

BlackBox
PUBLISHING & DISTRIBUTION

I am extremely grateful for two angels who I believe are always watching over me as shining stars!

DEDICATION

I am dedicating this book to three very special men who saved my life, and I could not have gotten through this breast cancer journey without them!

First, I am dedicating this book to Stu Jones, affectionately called Stu Dog, who was the father of one of my best friends and mentors, Fran Philip. Fran and I became fast friends when I first started working at L.L.Bean in 1996. Every weekend for four years, I skied Sunday River in Maine with Stu; his lovely wife, Vicky; Fran; her husband, George; and my husband at the time. Sometimes Sarah, Fran's sister, would visit and ski with the pack. We also sailed together in Maine, the British Virgin Islands, and the Grenadines. Stu became a close friend of mine, and occasionally called me his third daughter, which was a complete honor. He also nicknamed me Whoville, for Cindy Lou Who of *How the Grinch Stole Christmas!* It has stuck to this day, thirty-plus years later. Sadly, we lost Stu Dog on Thanksgiving of 2011, just before my diagnosis. It was at his memorial service and celebration of life that I received several strong messages from the universe and other friends to go see my doctor about the pain in my left breast. I believe Stu sent me these strong messages, which resulted in an early diagnosis of breast cancer, and is the reason I am still here today.

Second, I am dedicating this book to Dr. Keith Amos, who was my breast surgeon at University of North Carolina Hospital and Lineberger Cancer Center in Chapel Hill. Dr. Amos was an angel on this earth, and he never stopped caring for me. Dr. Amos was a realist who looked you straight in the eyes and told you exactly what he knew and that "everything was going to be OK." He gave me and my support team the belief and strength to carry on. He was available 24/7 and responded to every email or text promptly. He made himself available on weekends to take my calls and to talk me through treatments and surgery options. He introduced me to other women he treated that had similar situations. He always made me feel like I was his only patient, but I know he had hundreds of others. Sadly, Dr. Amos died suddenly and unexpectedly of an aortic aneurysm just three weeks after I became one year cancer free.

I am extremely grateful to my angels Stu Dog and Dr. Amos, who I believe are always watching over me as shining stars!

And finally, I dedicate this book to my best friend, lover, and fiancé, Craig Waller. I am eternally grateful and blessed to have found such a loving and caring partner. When I was diagnosed, Craig and I were newly in love and still developing our relationship. To his credit, Craig never let me down and always gave 150 percent of himself to take care of me, even when I was no fun to be around. I named him my Hot Male Nurse (HMN). According to Dr. Amos, many marriages do not survive cancer, especially breast cancer, because it is so shocking to lose your breasts. Craig wouldn't let that happen to us. He never gave up caring for me and loving me unconditionally. I remember Dr. Amos telling me one day, "You've got a keeper in Craig!" I am forever grateful for Craig and thank him from the bottom of my heart for being my primary supporter and caregiver. I love you, Craig, and cherish you with all my heart!

I am forever grateful for Craig and thank him from the bottom of my heart for being my primary supporter and caregiver. I LOVE YOU, Craig, and cherish you with all my heart!

CONTENTS

At the beginning of my journey,
I was told by my medical team
that I would become a changed
woman, for the better.
I didn't get it.

THE WOMAN WHO HAD IT ALL

At age forty-seven, I was healthy, vibrant, at the top of my game in the business world, and still turning heads with my long blond hair and lean glorious body. And then my world stopped in its tracks the day I was diagnosed with breast cancer. That was December 8, 2011, and here I am ten years later to share my story.

This book is about LOVE, family, and friends. It's about my journey and experience of beating breast cancer, or as I like to say, kicking it in the butt and "getting on it." It's also about sharing the many lessons I learned, to help others as they deal with life-threatening diseases like cancer. At the beginning of my journey, I was told by my medical team at UNC Chapel Hill—Dr. Keith Amos, Dr. Lisa Carey, and nurses Anna Kate Owen and Amy DePue—that I would become a changed woman, for the better. I looked at them like they had multiple heads. I didn't get it. I didn't understand how something so devastating could make me a better person. But I get it now, and that's why I want to share my journey with you. My life did change for the better from this experience. It was a hard lesson to learn something so simple and real, which is waking up each day being grateful for breathing, being alive, and living life.

My favorite saying while skiing is "get on it." I use it when everyone is standing around looking down a double black diamond slope like Black Hole at Sunday River, Maine, and no one moves because they are scared to ski it. "Get on it" is how I approached my breast cancer fight. I would attack, fall, get up, attack, fall, get up, and carry on with a positive attitude. Just like skiing a double black diamond—it's scary, challenging, frightening, and exhilarating. Eventually you reach the bottom of the run, then you reach the end. Maybe you lose an edge and fall the first time. But you get up, brush off the snow, and keep going. This is called having perseverance, which is a trait I didn't know I had until I dealt with breast cancer.

Thanks to my father for showing me how to be perseverant. I didn't do it alone. I had an incredible support system, which I called "my ring of power and circle of love." This circle of love started with my loving partner Craig, my family, and my friends. It expanded to my business colleagues, my incredible medical team, and my angels on earth and in heaven. I also learned how to have faith and to believe in God to carry me through this rough patch of life and walk beside me, like footprints in the sand.

I've always been a glass-half-full woman, but this eighteen-month journey and experience really tested my confidence, my strength, and my ability to remain positive. I am a changed woman for the better, and I want to inspire others to listen to the messages from the universe and to learn from them, like I did.

My intent is for this book is to help anybody that is dealing with sickness, disease, or heartache. It will be successful if I help at least one person learn how to cope and remain positive when life turns down a dark path. My hope is that my story will help you take away a new meaning of positivity and gain confidence, strength, and inspiration to deal with your daily journey of life! Breathe ON! SHINE ON!

A word of guidance for readers: the book's structure consists of two strands of narrative. My retelling of my story and reflections are within the chapters and have a white background. My journal appears throughout the book with grey-tinted pages. I decided to use entries from my journal for some of the key moments in the journey, as they convey a better sense of the immediacy and the real-time challenges as they arrived.

My goal for this book is that you, the reader, feel enlightened and uplifted by this "RING OF POWER AND CIRCLE OF LOVE."

The day your doctor
says those awful words,
"YOU HAVE CANCER,"
it shocks the seat
of your soul.

Chapter 1

EYES WIDE OPEN

When I look back on this time, I remember feeling like a deer in the headlights, frozen in time with shocked eyes and not sure where to turn or what to do. It all began in November of 2011, when I was living in Chapel Hill, NC. I was in the fourth month of a new position as the Chief Marketing Officer of the Specialty Retail division at Merkle, a database technology software company that focuses on helping retailers manage their customer and prospect data to drive revenue and profits. I was at the top of my business career and had built a successful personal brand for Cindy Marshall. I had no idea how my personal and business life would transform in one day—the day my doctor said, "You have cancer."

In early November, I had pain under my left armpit, near my left breast, but I didn't think much of it. It continued to bother me for three weeks, and I remember waking up in the middle of a deep sleep from the pain. I thought I slept wrong. I finally asked my manfriend and lover, Craig, to see if he felt anything under my left breast. Neither of us felt anything, but the pain didn't go away.

On November 23rd, the day before Thanksgiving, my best friend Fran's father passed away at seventy-eight years young. We called him Stu "Dog" Jones, and he was like a father to me. I admired and respected him with all my heart. We shared a special bond; he would often remind me that I was his third daughter, and that tickled me. He nicknamed me Whoville (for Cindy Lou Who) in 1996 when we first met, and this nickname is still holding today.

I share this loss with you because I believe Stu Dog had something to do with urging me to see my doctor in early December. It was at his funeral and celebration of life on December 3, 2011, that I received several strong messages to go see a doctor. Stu's celebration of life was in South Freeport, Maine, at the home of Fran and George, and it was there that I spoke with two friends, Shawn and Liz, who were both battling cancer. I shared with them my silly breast pain that I'd had for a month and told them I didn't think it was anything. I was always told that breast cancer didn't hurt, you can't feel it, and it doesn't cause pain. This is not always true; breast cancer can hurt. Shawn and Liz encouraged me to see a doctor. That night, I shared a room with a good friend, Kim, and she told me the same thing: "Don't mess with this and call your doctor first thing on Monday!"

On Monday, December 5th, I called my OBGYN, Dr. Mezzer, in Greensboro, NC, which is where I lived when I first moved to North Carolina two years earlier. I was given an appointment two days later, Wednesday, December 7th. I really liked this doctor a lot, so I kept him when I moved to Chapel Hill. He gave me a physical exam and said the words I pray you never have to hear: "Yes, I feel something, and I want you to get a mammogram and ultrasound."

I thought, *What??? NO way . . . this can't be happening to me.* I responded with, "OK, I will go today if they can take me, but I am flying to California tomorrow for work meetings and a mini vacation with Craig." I was determined not to let anyone down on the business front, plus I was in denial.

Immediately after my physical exam, I went to the Breast Center of Greensboro Imaging on my doctor's orders. It was only 11 a.m., and I thought to myself, *OK, this is precautionary. I don't have anything wrong, plus I have a lot of work to do.* I was seen right away for a mammogram scan. I was shuttled back and forth in my "Johnny gown" between imaging rooms and waiting rooms until finally, the doctor was ready to see me. Dr. Boyle turned out to be extremely handsome and very easy on the eyes. That made me smile! Dr. Dreamy—my nickname for him—said to me, "Yes, we see some cysts; in fact, four of them. Three at two o'clock and one at two thirty," explaining their positions with reference to the hands on a clock. "The large one is of concern because it has irregular edges," he said. "We need to take a closer look with an ultrasound to confirm." Two nurses got me settled and one held my hand as Dr. Dreamy started his procedure.

He showed me four spots that looked like tumors. One was the size of a quarter, one a dime, one a nickel, and one the size of a pencil eraser. He wanted to biopsy them. I was now freaking out! I called Craig at work, but he couldn't get away. I decided to proceed, still thinking I had to get on the plane in the morning for California. The nurses prepared the skin and got me set up for the biopsy. Dr. Dreamy injected me with Novocaine, and we waited a few minutes before he started the needle biopsy.

We had complications. The first time he went in, using the ultrasound machine as a guide, he went very deep, and I could feel it. I started screaming in pain so awful, I can remember the pain to this day. They realized I was not numb enough and had to give me more Novocaine! *WHAT??* Now I was in tears and scared. The second time, I was even more nervous, knowing what to expect, but luckily there was no pain, and he took the four needle biopsies and inserted a titanium chip to identify the location for tracking purposes. Eight needles total.

I was crying and in total shock with my eyes wide open. They told me to go home, put ice on the biopsy spot, and cancel my trip. They sent the biopsies to the lab and informed me the lead doctor would call me that evening. I called Craig in tears, and he told me to go home to rest up. I was not convinced I needed to cancel my business trip until Craig talked sense into me. It was pouring rain as I drove home to Chapel Hill, an hour away. I cried hard the entire time. Craig arrived later to hold and love me as we both cried.

The doctor called me that night to say she would like to see me in the morning, and to bring a friend. Now we were both scared and didn't know what to think. Thursday, December 8th, arrived. At 9:00 a.m., Craig and I met with the lead doctor at the Breast Center of Greensboro. She was very calming but also very direct. She said the three words I never wanted to hear, "You have cancer." I was diagnosed with invasive ductal carcinoma, with four tumors totaling over two centimeters. I was told I had very aggressive, fast-growing malignant breast cancer in my left breast. We didn't know the source of the cancer, what they call markers, so they couldn't tell me what stage it was. What we did know was that it was growing fast, because I had a clean mammogram nine months earlier.

My thoughts were racing. *How can this be? I thought cancer moved slower. I didn't think cancer hurt. What do I do now??* Lots of questions and no answers.

Next, they scheduled two appointments for Monday, December 12th—one for an MRI with Greensboro Imaging, and one with the breast surgeon at the Breast Center of Greensboro. Craig took me home and held me, and we cried. We were both in shock.

Sharing the news with my family brought my fears to the forefront. I kept thinking, *Now it's my turn . . . and I will survive, I will beat this! Remain positive.* Craig had a Christmas party on Thursday night, so he built a nice fire for me. I sat by the fire to make my calls. It was not easy. I started with Fran, who was extremely helpful, being a ten-year breast cancer survivor. I called my family and my close girlfriends. Lots of tears that night were soothed by many hugs from Craig and Poppy, his dog.

What did Cindy do? What I always do—I persevered and carried on. I pushed forward like this was a business problem I had to solve. The next day, I decided it was time to network and get second opinions. Like a good leader, I researched my options. I called everyone I knew for referrals and made calls all day. Several people suggested Duke, and a few UNC Chapel Hill. I called both hospitals to get appointments. I had the name of a great doctor at UNC, and that helped me get an appointment for the following week.

Now it's my turn . . .
and I will survive, I will beat this!
Remain positive.

I was raised to be strong, confident, honest, compassionate, brave, and driven. I was given everything a little girl would want, except a sister, but I had many girlfriends and a vivid imagination.

Chapter 2

MEET CINDY LOU WHO

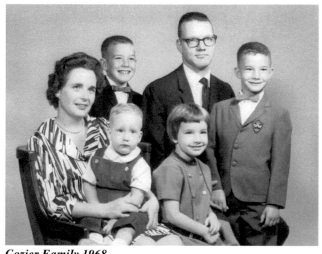

Cozier Family 1968

Before I continue, I need to share more about my background for context. All I ever dreamed of as a child was an ordinary life. From the time I had my first doll, I knew I wanted to become a mother and a wife. I loved to play homemaker and mother, especially with my massive Barbie doll collection. Plus, I loved to help my mother with household chores and cooking. I wanted to be just like her. I always looked up to my mother with pride and joy. When I look back on my childhood, I feel very blessed to have been raised by incredibly loving parents, to have known all four of my grandparents, to have three amazing brothers, to have grown up with many animals (dogs, gerbils, parakeets, and turtles), and to have experienced an extended family with more than sixty cousins.

During my cancer treatment, and even earlier in my career, many people asked me where my strength came from. I believe it's from my brilliant family heritage, my parents' unconditional love, growing up with three brothers, and my adventurous childhood experiences. I think it's important to share some of my childhood, so you have a better understanding of where my foundation came from.

Who is Cindy Lou Who? My birth name is Cynthia Jane Cozier, but my nickname is Cindy Lou Who, or Whoville. My parents were raised in the Midwest. My mother was from Indianapolis, Indiana, and my father from Cleveland, Ohio. Mom was raised on a working farm with horses, cattle, pigs, dogs, cats, and lots of cornfields. She was the youngest of five children, with ten years between my mother and her next oldest sister. She went to public schools and was a very smart student who loved to read and win spelling bees. My father was raised in the suburbs of Cleveland known as Shaker Heights and brought up in an upper class, very strict household. He was required to wear a coat and tie to dinner every night. He had a maid and a gardener, and he was the oldest of three children. My father was sent away for high school to Proctor Academy, a private boarding school in New Hampshire. That was where he first played baseball and learned to become a confident young man.

I am number three of four children, all brothers, so you can only imagine where some of my strength comes from. My brothers and I were brought up in a middle-class Presbyterian family. We went to church every Sunday and were required to sit down to dinner by six p.m. sharp. There were many household rules to abide by, but we were also given freedom to enjoy life the way it's meant to be lived as children. We spent a lot of time outdoors because we didn't have computers or phones. We loved to play kick the can, capture the flag, touch football, hide and seek, and many other neighborhood games.

I was born in Corvallis, OR, while my dad was studying forestry at Oregon State University. When I was two years old, Dad got a job in the Forestry Service in Juneau, AK, so we picked up and moved. Rich, the oldest, was seven, and Dave was six. At the time, Mom was five months pregnant, and my younger brother, JD, short for John Daniel, was born in May of 1966, just four months later. I don't remember much about Juneau other than living on a frozen lake. I have one memory of Alaska, which was looking out the window to watch my mother and brothers ice skating on the lake. Then Dad began yelling because he saw my mother fall and my brothers bringing her back on the sled—she broke her arm! I remember my brothers telling me how much they loved Alaska because there was so much snow all winter long and many snow days.

The next thirteen years of my life were spent in Potomac, MD, in suburban neighborhoods. I have very fond memories of my childhood in Potomac, and especially the love that was shown to me by my parents. We lived in three different homes, but the one I remember most was Weatherwood Court in Country Place. It had a very large oak tree in the middle of the driveway. I learned to ride a bike by riding around the tree a hundred times with training wheels on! We could walk to school and had tons of friends. Everyone played sports and participated in the church youth groups. We were members of a tennis and swim club, which I frequented during the summer months with my girlfriends. We even had a rock 'n' roll band practice in our basement during my junior high years, thanks to my brother, Rich, who managed the band and was a rock 'n' roll fanatic. The basement was equipped with a pool table that saw endless hours of competition. My brothers would build models of military tanks, planes, ships, and model diorama scenes complete with mountains, lakes, and railroad tracks used to recreate different battle scenes.

My childhood gave me a solid foundation and strong belief system. It comes from an incredibly deep and rich heritage on both sides of my family. My parents taught us to be kind, honest, loving, and respectful of one another. I can still hear my mother saying to me over and over, "Honesty is the best policy. Whatever action you make will always come back to you, so be honest in everything you do." That has always stuck with me, but there were times I was not always honest with myself, especially when it came to taking care of myself. Another one of my mother's favorite sayings was "Always treat others as you wish to be treated, with respect."

I was raised to be strong, confident, honest, compassionate, brave, and driven. I was given everything a little girl would want, except a sister, but I had many girlfriends and a vivid imagination. I loved *The Brady Bunch* so much that I decided to have an imaginary sister, Jan Brady of *The Brady Bunch!* On the masculine side, I loved being a tomboy, trying to keep up with my three brothers, and playing with Hot Wheels, LEGOs, and trains. On the feminine side, I played with Barbie dolls, stuffed animals, Suzy Homemaker, Twister, Operation, and Prize Property. I also learned to be a caretaker of the family while I assisted my mother in the kitchen or cleaning the house. As I became a teenager, rock 'n' roll was the most important part of everyday life, including spending hours at Peaches record store and making wish lists of new albums I wanted for Christmas or my birthday. We were a driven family and the kids were expected to finish high school in four years and go straight to college to finish in four years.

During my childhood years, we traveled to approximately forty out of the fifty states by car, all before I was sixteen years old. Every summer, we planned a two- to three-week vacation that centered around Presbyterian Mariners Cruises. No, not a boat cruise, but a week-long fellowship gathering for Presbyterians nationwide. We would load up the Ford station wagon and drive to the conference locations at universities across America—in Kansas, Missouri, Colorado, Nebraska, and California, to name a few. Mom was always organized with a travel itinerary that included lodging at church hostels (families that opened their homes to us) or an occasional hotel, tourist attractions with scenic drives, and visits with our vast family around America. It was truly an experience that my siblings and I looked forward to each summer. We developed deep friendships with other church children and became pen pals during the following year.

The Mariner conference events were only one week long, but it was an amazing and memorable week. As children, we were separated from our parents in different parts of the campus with our activities, while our parents had their own activities, such as bible study. We always shared meals and fellowship time with our parents, including singing church songs with hundreds of people outside in scenic

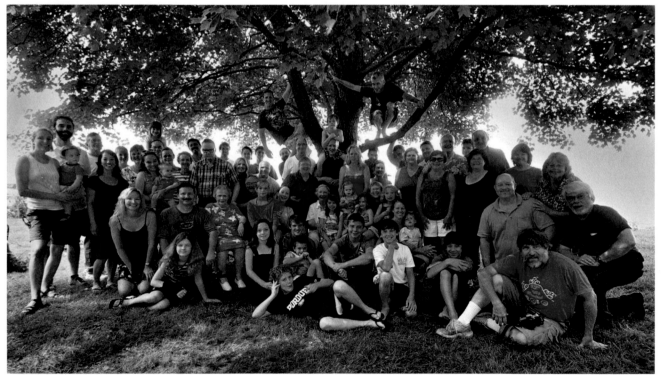

Glossbrenner Extended Family July 2011

locations. It was magical. This was such a memorable experience for me, and I truly believe it's one of the reasons I am so driven and so confident in my daily life. There is one experience I will never forget that I want to share with you.

One night at a campfire event, eating s'mores, we sat around singing and holding hands. One of the counselors had an acoustic guitar, and he guided us into moments of silence and asked us to open our hearts and minds to the universe above (to think about what Jesus Christ meant to us and who God was to us) and it was an extremely moving experience. It was during one of these silent moments that I received a strong message: "You are an old soul. You have lived many times before and you were put on this earth to love and teach others." I didn't know what this meant at the time, but maybe it was what drove me subconsciously to become a successful woman in retail leadership. I've learned over the years to be more open to hearing and listening to my inner voice, my intuition. I have a deep intuition, and when I open my crown chakra and listen, I feel calm and at peace. Everyone has intuition, but we need to learn how to hear it and listen to it.

EVERYONE has intuition, but we need to learn how to hear it and listen to it.

My doctor proceeded to tell me my only option was to have surgery right away to remove my breast.

Chapter 3

SHOCK SETS IN

Back to my cancer journey . . .

On December 12th, I had my first consult with a surgeon in Greensboro. I woke up with a sinus infection, which didn't help at all! This is my weak spot, my Achilles' heel. Now I had to see my primary care doctor to get antibiotics for the sinus problem.

I was so strong until the end of the day. The doctor's visit was overwhelming, with so much information, so many options, and no new news. Craig and Linh, one of my good friends and work colleagues, joined me at the doctor's, and this helped a lot. The MRI was scheduled from 6:45 to 7:45 p.m., and Linh waited with me. Once the IV was inserted, I lay flat on the machine, breasts down. The machine made very loud noises, like a jackhammer or shotguns. At least I had ear plugs and music to listen to. It didn't hurt but was very strange. The noise the was worst part.

I was so hungry that I went to Panera for comfort food, a panini to go. I wasn't thinking straight and walked straight into the glass door at Panera and got a huge welt on my forehead! All I could do was cry. *How much more can I take?* I thought. *Can I drive home to Chapel Hill?* I managed to drive and had a good chat with my brother JD along the way. When I got home, my girlfriends from Vermont sent love pictures in pink, which helped cheer me up.

The results were sent to the Breast Center of Greensboro and to UNC Chapel Hill. I met with the breast surgeon in Greensboro as planned. He read me the results of the MRI, which told him that the cancer was now more than double in size. It was over five centimeters, because it was in my ducts and had moved all the way to my nipple. I was in shock. *How can this be?* I wondered. *Why did the mammogram not see this?* When I posed these questions to the doctor, he told me that MRIs pick up more detail, and mammos only identify the problem but don't show everything. He proceeded to tell me my only option was to have surgery right away to remove my breast. *Are you serious? WTF? How can this be? NO!!* I couldn't think, I couldn't focus. By this time, I really wanted my second opinion, which happened to be the next day with UNC Chapel Hill.

In addition to Craig as my primary caretaker, I now had Mary Sullivan in my life as my "angel on earth." Mary is a longtime friend of Stu Dog and Vicky (Fran's stepmother) and lives in Chapel Hill. Craig and Mary joined me for my first appointment at UNC. We met with Dr. Lisa Carey, who became my oncologist; my nurses Anna Kate Owen and Amy DePue; and Dr. Keith Amos, who became my breast surgeon. Mary was amazing and took all the notes so that Craig and I could listen to the doctors. The doctors were direct and to the point, but also very calming. They discussed the results of the Greensboro biopsies and MRI. They explained their process of getting more tests at UNC to validate everything.

That meant more mammograms, another biopsy *(NO!)*, and an MRI. I really didn't want to do these tests again, but I had to trust their process. Mary drove me to each appointment and held my hand during every procedure. She told me to go to my happy place. That's what I did. I would imagine fields of sunflowers and fields of lavender in Provence. This made me smile! Each time I had a test, off I went to Provence to see the lovely yellow and purple fields of light and love.

I started the UNC testing process one week after I was first diagnosed. Mary picked me up at 9:00 a.m., and I wasn't home until 5:00 p.m. The morning was slow. The mammo didn't get done until 11:00, even though it was scheduled at 9:30. I had another ultrasound. This time, UNC found a large mass at six o'clock on my left breast (the fifth one to be identified). My poor breast was very swollen and painful. I finally saw the genetics team at 1:00 p.m., the nurse at 3:00 p m., and Dr. Amos, my breast surgeon, at 4:00 p.m. No news other than the new lump. Now I needed another biopsy! Ugh! UNC needed their own MRI report and full pathology report as a baseline. They also wanted to find out what type of receptor I had (estrogen, progesterone, or HER2), which would take a few weeks. The best news was that I received approval from UNC to take my two-week vacation to Ireland and London for Christmas, my birthday, and New Year's! Yippee!! I could relax until my next appointment on January 4, 2012.

I can't forget all the reading material. During these two weeks, I started to read everything the doctors gave me, including a large book from Greensboro and another one from UNC. There was so much information and noise online about breast cancer, but I chose not to listen to those opinions. I quickly become a student of breast cancer and read as much as I could. It was overwhelming and scary at the same time. I was still in shock and not sure what to do, except to listen to my doctors.

Are you serious?
WTF?
How can this be?
NO!!

My first position was as a marketing coordinator for *Bicycle Guide* and *Ultrasport* magazines.

Chapter 4

THE ROLLER COASTER OF MY LOVE LIFE AND CAREER

A little more on my adult background. As a driven individual, I went directly from college to work. My first position was as a marketing coordinator for *Bicycle Guide* and *Ultrasport* magazines, part of Raben Publishing in Boston, MA. During my two and a half years at Raben, I learned how to lead PR events, sell advertising space, support a sales team, prepare analysis, gather insights from the analysis, and launch a magazine from scratch, *The Walking Magazine*. I loved my first job, and I loved networking, which led me to my second position as a circulation manager at *Inc.* magazine, responsible for their subscription solicitation. In this role, I learned about renting mailing lists and measuring the success or failure of them. I learned how to be part of a team and contribute in a meaningful way. I made some close friends and had my first mentor at *Inc.* magazine. They taught me that work CAN be fun, especially when we would take an afternoon off to celebrate a success by going sailing as a team. In both positions, I learned how to use my right and left brain, which soon became one of my greatest strengths. I was able to analyze data with actionable insights as well as deliver compelling brand messaging.

Meanwhile, on the personal front, I had moved in with my college sweetheart after we graduated. We were engaged and married four years later, when I was only twenty-four. We had the dream wedding I always wanted with 150 people at National Presbyterian Church in Washington, DC, followed by an elegant reception and celebration at a large mansion in Maryland. Life was right on track. My Barbie dolls would have been happy!

I continued to climb the ladder, got promoted, and made more money. We bought our first house in Marshfield, MA, so I decided to get a job closer to home in Hingham, MA, a fifteen-minute commute. Now I was a Director of Marketing for DM Management, a direct marketing company that had four catalog brands, one being J.Jill. We bought a larger home overlooking the ocean in Marshfield. My husband got anther job that took him overseas for months at a time. That was when we started to drift apart. About five years into our marriage, I learned he was having an affair. I was devastated. We had been thinking of starting a family. He agreed to see a marriage counselor. We tried three different ones, but it didn't work. It became very clear that he didn't want to leave the relationship with the other woman, so I decided to leave him. We agreed to separate, then divorced a year later.

My heart was completely broken, and my dreams were shattered. I asked myself, *How do I start again?* It was time to leave the south shore of Boston. I chatted with several recruiters and started interviewing. I landed a great position as Vice President of Marketing for a larger retailer and cataloger, Appleseed's. I was twenty-nine years old and had achieved my goal of becoming a VP before thirty! This new position helped me focus and carry on with a broken heart. I moved to Marblehead, MA, which was ten minutes from my new office in Beverly. I didn't socialize for six months as I focused on my new role and poured my heart and soul into it. Finally, I decided to get out and meet people in Marblehead, so I joined a Wednesday night sailing group. This was the best thing I did to move on personally. I met a new girlfriend, who became one of my besties. I ran into many college friends that I had lost touch with. Now, I was laughing again and enjoying being on the water! Eight of us decided to rent a ski house in Sugarbush, VT, that winter. It was so much fun that we did it for three years total. It was a complete blast and just what I needed to start dating again. I dated a few men, but no one that set my heart on fire.

Two years into my new life in Marblehead, I met a man at a sailing party, and he took my breath away. We became instant friends after many hours chatting that weekend. He lived in Connecticut and was a professional sailor who was ten years older than me. He was thoughtful, caring, kind, and handsome. He had recently lost his wife of five years to cancer three months earlier and was still grieving. He was a heartfelt and loving man who took the time to send a dozen roses to my office! I was smitten! We quickly developed a relationship and our love blossomed. We were engaged four months later at Sugarbush Resort while skiing in the back woods. It was very romantic. I had been keeping a journal after my first marriage split up, and I had written down what I wanted in a man. He fit the mold. I had no doubt this was the right person for me and my dreams were being answered. I also felt divine intervention from his late wife. It was as though she chose us to be together.

We got married a year later in Kiawah Island, NC, in a small wedding with family and close friends. I become a stepmother of two beautiful children, Christopher and Elizabeth, who were eleven and thirteen at the time. Life had turned around for me and I was happy. His business took him to Portland, ME, to run an America's Cup program for the 2000 cup in Auckland, New Zealand. I needed to find a position in Maine. This time, I networked with my industry contacts at L.L.Bean during a six-month stretch. Persistence paid off and I landed a role as Manager of Loyalty Marketing running the L.L.Bean Visa credit card program that was recently launched. We bought a house in the woods of Durham, ME, and moved in with our dog Brie and cat Winnie. We made a lot of new friends, some that would become lifelong friends, like Fran, George, Vicky, Stu, and Sarah. We loved it there.

My career progressed with L.L.Bean, and I was asked to lead marketing and brand design for the launch of a new women's apparel brand, Freeport Studio. My husband was doing great raising money and preparing for the 1999 Louis Vuitton racing series in Auckland. This was the pre-race to determine who would race against the New Zealand team for the America's Cup. The America's Cup ended, and now it was time to find another job. The dot-com boom had taken off, and we both wanted to chase it. We found roles in two different startup dot-com businesses in North Adams, MA. We bought a home on a hundred acres in Williamstown, MA, and we immersed ourselves in this new country lifestyle. Again, we made many new friends and loved living there. Then the dot-com bust happened, and we got restless and fearful of losing our jobs, so we both landed positions in Rhode Island and moved again in 2001. I became the VP of Marketing for Ross-Simons, a $250 million jewelry brand that had seventeen retail stores. I was very grateful for the time I spent at eZiba.com, because it was an eighteen-month crash course in digital marketing, just like completing a two-year MBA!

After renting for a year, we built a home in North Kingstown. Life was an adventure and a challenge for us in Rhode Island. He was traveling all the time, sailing, and working, while I had a lot of pressure at work. I wanted children but soon learned that he didn't. This caused a lot of tension in our marriage. I decided to see a counselor to help me through it. After all, that was my childhood dream, and I was about to turn forty. I finally accepted that I wouldn't have children and was grateful to love my two fabulous stepchildren, five amazing nieces and nephews, and a marketing team that needed nurturing and teaching. I would focus on enjoying life with my husband. After three years living there, his job was not going well, and I was ready for a change. We decided to leave the area, and I started searching for another position.

This time, I didn't rush the process. I wanted to find a company that was a great fit, where I loved the people, the products, and the location. I ended up at the Vermont Country Store as Head of Marketing, Brand, and Ecommerce. We moved to Shaftsbury, VT, which was halfway between my new office in Manchester Center and our good friends in Williamstown, MA. We bought a lovely farmhouse with almost twenty acres of land. It was a large home to take care of, but we loved the view and the land. During the five years we lived there, my husband didn't work, so I was supporting the household. I was fine with this if he was taking care of the house. He was still sailing domestically and in Europe, which would take him away for months at a time. He was also an avid cyclist and president of a local cycling club. He was playing hard, and I was working hard. It wasn't working for me, and I was drained. We ended up growing apart, and I was angry having to work late and take care of the house while he was off playing. Sadly, we separated and eventually divorced after I left Vermont for a new role as a president of a wedding business in Greensboro, NC. That is how I came to live in North Carolina.

This time, I didn't rush the process. I wanted to find a company that was a great fit, where I loved the people, the products, and the location.

We learned that I had what was called "triple negative metastatic ductal carcinoma, stage 2B." *Still Greek to me—what does this mean?*

Chapter 5

LET GO AND HAVE FUN!

B ack to my cancer journey . . .
After I finished the first set of tests at UNC, we met with Dr. Amos and Dr. Carey on December 18th to learn about my breast cancer markers, which would indicate where the cancer came from and what the possible treatments were. Craig, Mary, and I met with the doctors again, and Mary was our scribe. We learned that I had what was called "triple negative metastatic ductal carcinoma, stage 2B." *Still Greek to me—what does this mean?* Triple negative means it did not come from estrogen, progesterone, or HER2—basically the skin cells (human epidermal growth factor receptor 2). Triple negative tends to occur more often in younger women and in women who are African American or Hispanic/Latina. It is a very fast-growing cancer and harder to treat because you can't use hormone therapy like Tamoxifen. It was stage 2B because we caught it early enough. The triple negative part made it a B and not an A because it was fast growing (there are only A and B between stages).

Why does the marker matter? Dr. Amos said, "Because you have triple negative, we know you HAVE to have chemo; there is no choice. It is the most aggressive form of breast cancer, and it grows fast. What we don't know is if the cancer has spread to the rest of your body." They wanted to schedule a lymph node test for the beginning of January, so we booked that on January 9th. They also wanted me to get a BRCA test, which is the genetic testing that tells you if you have a gene mutation for breast cancer in your cells, meaning it could be hereditary. We had already done a family tree to see who else in my family had any sort of cancer, and because there were over five instances, they suggested this. They also wanted one more scan of my right breast just to be sure there was no cancer there.

It was December 18th, and I was leaving for Ireland and England on the 20th for two weeks. I wanted to go on holiday. I asked if it was OK to travel and Dr. Amos said, "Go have fun and enjoy the last two weeks of the year. That won't change anything, but let's meet on January 4th when the balance of the results come back, and we can work on a final treatment plan."

"Are you sure?" I asked.

"Yes," he said "GO!" I felt better and decided that was exactly what I would do! But before I could leave, I had one more scan of my right breast, the clean one.

Off I went to Ireland for Christmas to be with one of my best friends, Daria, and her family near Shannon. We had a spectacular time, and the love was overwhelming! I remember crying at the Christmas Eve service at their local church in downtown Quin. It was very moving as I prayed to live to sing Christmas songs again.

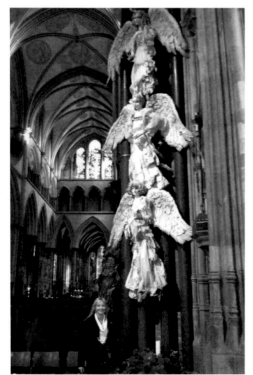

Me with Angels of Salisbury!

On the 26th, I flew to London to meet Craig and celebrate my birthday with his best friends in Godalming. We laughed a lot and celebrated life!

We went to Salisbury to visit Craig's mother, Jeanne, which was the first time I had met her in person. We toured the Salisbury Cathedral, which took my breath away! It was a very moving experience. I prayed to the angels to help me heal and give me the ability to cope. They heard me.

London was amazing! We were lucky to stay at the Four Seasons, one of Craig's clients, which was a once-in-a-lifetime experience. We toured downtown London and did a champagne tour of the London Eye. Truly magnificent! On New Year's Eve, we watched the fireworks from the tenth floor of the Four Seasons! So beautiful and romantic!

This was exactly what the doctor ordered. I forgot about

everything for at least ten days—it was perfect! Then January 1st came, and I was a complete wreck. The shock was over, and now fear had set in! I was so worried and not sure what to expect when I returned home on January 2nd. I had no idea how I would cope with everything.

Back to the business side of my life. Four months prior to my diagnosis, I had taken a position as Chief Marketing Officer (CMO) for a smaller division of Merkle, a large database marketing company. I was excited about this opportunity, not only to learn their strategic insights, thought leadership, and innovative technology, but to work with many of their retail brands. When I was diagnosed, I decided not to tell my employer until I knew more about my prognosis and treatment, which would be revealed at the big meeting on January 4, 2012. It turned out that was a wise decision.

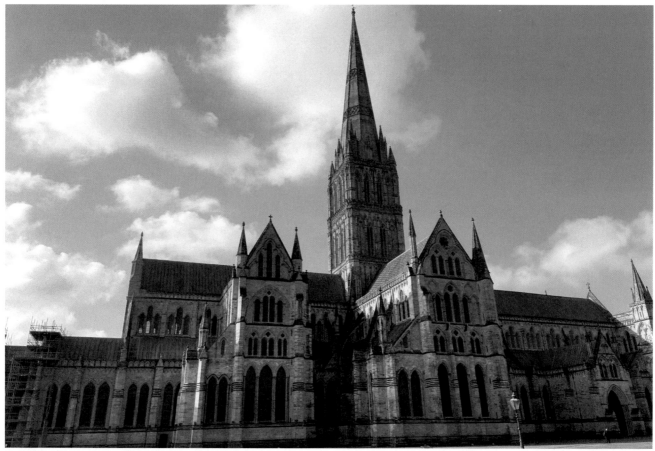

Salisbury Cathedral, England, December 2011

Will I be strong enough?
How can I focus on my health
and work at the same time?
What will the future bring?
How will my boss react when
I tell him about my cancer?

Chapter 6

THE FEAR IS REAL

We got home to North Carolina on January 2nd from the UK. I was completely exhausted. Craig and I went back to our separate homes in Chapel Hill and Greensboro.

I was now completely freaking out inside. I was so scared about life and what the next few months would bring. My thoughts were all over the place. *Will I be strong enough? How can I focus on my health and work at the same time? I am grateful to have Craig in my life, but I also live alone—can I cope? What will the future bring? I don't love my job, but now is not the time to find a new position. How will my boss react when I tell him about my cancer? What does the future hold? I am happy that Fran is coming to visit to help with doctors; she knows what to do.*

Our big meeting with all the doctors was set for January 4th, which was the day I would learn about my treatment plan. Fran, a breast cancer survivor and thriver, arrived on the 3rd to support me for the big reveal. It was so great to have her support, especially because she understands breast cancer, having been there before. I had never known fear like this. I was so afraid of the pain, afraid of dying, afraid of losing my breasts, afraid of the uncertain future. I couldn't stand it. Part of my childhood taught me to always be strong in front of others and not break down. This was the bad part of being brought up so strong and confident—it was hard to be weak and give in. Bottom line, I was holding a lot of the pain and fear inside me, which was tearing me apart.

Fran and I went upstairs to prepare for bed and I completely lost it; I couldn't stop crying. I kept saying, "I am so afraid!"

Fran asked, "What are you afraid of?"

I answered, "The pain, I'm afraid of dying, the unknown, losing my breasts, losing my job."

Fran, in her strong leadership voice, said, "Cindy, there is no reason to be afraid! Fear is fear itself. All you have to do is step on it, and it will go away!"

She hugged me and held me while I cried. I will never forget that moment. It helped me understand that it's OK to cry, it's OK to feel the feelings, and it's OK to be fearful. This stayed with me throughout the entire journey. Whenever I felt fear creeping up, my mantra was "Fear is fear itself. Let it go," and that is what I did.

Not only is Fran one of my best friends, but she was also a mentor to me in the professional world when we worked together. I've learned a lot from Fran. Now that I had the fear behind me, it was time to face the doctors and my treatment plan.

FEAR is fear itself. All you have to do is step on it, and it will go away!

CHEMO?

Sixteen weeks?

What do I need to know?

How will I survive this?

Chapter 7

THE DECISION TREE

Craig, Fran, Mary, and I headed to UNC Chapel Hill on January 4th to meet with Dr. Carey and Dr. Amos to discuss my options. We were informed that I had no choice and needed to have chemotherapy first. I was diagnosed with triple negative breast cancer, which is one of the most aggressive kinds of breast cancer. They prescribed eight treatments over sixteen weeks, basically one week on and one week off. The chemo was Adriamycin, aka the red devil. There were also five other chemo drugs, but I can't remember all the names. I do recall the Taxol was first, because that is the most intense one, and they wanted to start me off with the strongest first.

We were all in shock, but mostly me and Craig. *Chemo? Sixteen weeks? What do I need to know? How will I survive this?* I had visions of movies with people throwing up all day, pale faced, drained, bony, and very sick. I didn't want this . . . why me? I was so angry and so scared, but it was Dr. Amos that made all of us feel better.

I will always remember Dr. Amos staring me in the eyes with a calm and loving face to tell me, "We know you need chemotherapy, so there is no concern right now about what type of surgery to have. Let's start the chemo and then re-image you halfway through to see if it's being effective. This will give you two months to start thinking about surgery. In the meantime, we need to determine if the cancer is in your lymph nodes, so we need to remove some nodes under your left arm." It was all so matter of fact, like a boss telling me what to do, but with compassion and love. He was absolutely the best possible doctor that anyone could ask for. Looking back on it now, I realize how lucky I was to be living in

Chapel Hill, NC, with a five-minute drive to UNC Chapel Hill Cancer Center.

There is a saying in yoga by Hafiz: "The place where you are right now God circled on a map for you. Wherever your eyes and arms and heart can move against the earth and sky, the beloved has bowed there. The beloved has bowed there knowing you were coming." I believe that is exactly what happened. God moved me to North Carolina because he wanted me to meet Craig, to be close to my parents in Asheville, and to be close to UNC Chapel Hill when it was time for treatment. I believe in the spirits of the universe, and I know my angels and God circled on a map my temporary home in Chapel Hill.

After I knew my diagnosis and treatment plan, it was time to tell my boss. I reached out on January 5th to tell him. He was compassionate and understanding. A week later, he called to tell me my position was being eliminated. The parent company didn't want to have two CMO roles, so my position was being eliminated and I was being moved to a strategic services division. I didn't care at that point—all I was focused on was my breast cancer, whether I was going to die, and how would I move forward. I used to let my work rule my life. Now, I was focused on my health and nothing else mattered.

After I knew my diagnosis and treatment plan, it was time to tell my boss. I reached out on January 5th to tell him. He was compassionate and understanding. A week later, he called to tell me my position was being eliminated.

Fran was a Godsend to me for many reasons. First, she put her business mind on and calmly told me not to get overwhelmed about the decisions. "Let's make a decision tree," she said. This was brilliant! It allowed me to shift from fear and anger to visualizing a picture of what my choices were with the possible outcomes. I prayed on this visual that I wouldn't have cancer in my lymph nodes so I wouldn't need radiation, and most importantly, that it had not metastasized. I prayed that we caught it early.

By now, the cards filled with love were pouring in from all my family and friends. This is something my friend Lois sent me, which I love!

"Don't worry about ANYTHING but in all your prayers ask God for what you need, ALWAYS asking him with a THANKFUL heart and God's peace which is far beyond human understanding will keep your heart and mind SAFE in union with Jesus Christ. My friends, fill your minds with those things that are GOOD and deserve PRAISE, things that are true, noble, right, pure, lovely, and honorable."

Philippians 4:6–8

My Breast Cancer Decision Tree

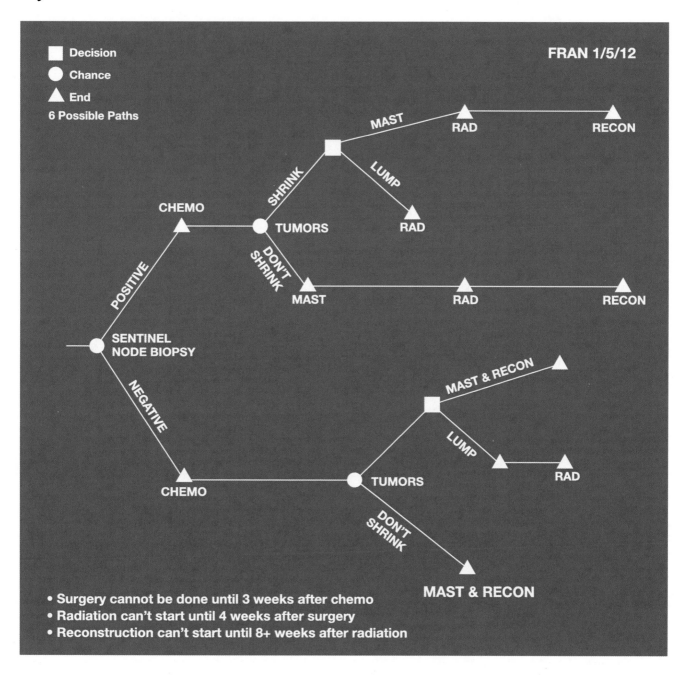

When I was at my lowest,
love from my friends carried
me through.

Chapter 8

FOREVER GRATEFUL

When I was at my lowest point, it was the love and support of my friends that carried me through. I was so moved by the outpouring of support I received. So much so, that it actually became overwhelming to communicate with everyone! That's when Fran suggested I create a page on the CaringBridge website. I didn't want to do this. I didn't want to have everything public. Fran, the wiser one, created it anyway. She knew I would need it, and for that I am forever grateful. First, I learned it didn't have to be public. I chose who was invited. Second, it became my release, the way I let go of the pain and the fear. Finally, the response I received from my network of family and friends blew my mind. The outpouring of love, caring, and compassion was amazing. I had no idea how much I meant to everyone, and their love helped me through this tough period of life. It was truly remarkable. During the six months I was going through treatment, I had close to 8,000 visitors to my CaringBridge journal. When I needed it again nine months later, it grew to over 9,000 visitors!

This was my journal.

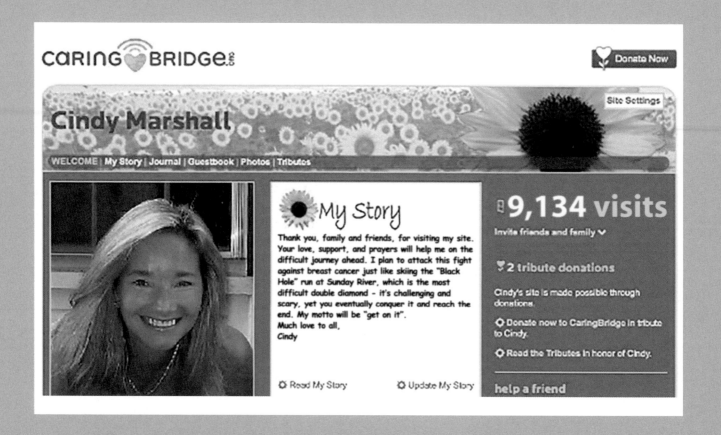

CARING BRIDGE.org

Donate Now

Cindy Marshall

Site Settings

WELCOME | My Story | Journal | Guestbook | Photos | Tributes

My Story

Thank you, family and friends, for visiting my site. Your love, support, and prayers will help me on the difficult journey ahead. I plan to attack this fight against breast cancer just like skiing the "Black Hole" run at Sunday River, which is the most difficult double diamond - it's challenging and scary, yet you eventually conquer it and reach the end. My motto will be "get on it".
Much love to all,
Cindy

Read My Story   Update My Story

9,134 visits

Invite friends and family ⌄

2 tribute donations

Cindy's site is made possible through donations.

Donate now to CaringBridge in tribute to Cindy.

Read the Tributes in honor of Cindy.

help a friend

Introduction from my CaringBridge site:

Thank you, family and friends, for visiting my site. Your love, support, and prayers will help me on the difficult journey ahead. I plan to attack this fight against breast cancer just like skiing the "Black Hole" run at Sunday River, which is the most difficult double diamond—it's challenging and scary, yet you eventually conquer it and reach the end. My motto will be GET ON IT.

Background Story

I was diagnosed with breast cancer on December 8. Since then, I have been through a whirlwind of various tests and procedures to correctly diagnose the extent of the cancer and the protocol to treat it.

Now all the test results are in and there is lots of good news to celebrate. The genetic testing was negative, as was the core biopsy on the right side and the sentinel node biopsy on the left side. Yippee!!!

On to chemotherapy, which starts January 20 and runs for sixteen weeks—a total of eight treatments, one every two weeks. About halfway through, they will check to see if the tumors are shrinking. After chemo, it will be time to think about surgery, but right now I am just focused on the next sixteen weeks and choosing the right wardrobe of wigs to express the many sides of my personality!

I am fortunate to have a super Team Cindy at UNC Cancer Hospital in Chapel Hill. The doctors and their staffs are all fabulous—I know I'm in great hands.

My friends and family have been an amazing rock for me so far, and I know that I could not go on this journey without them. Thank you for all your support and visiting my site to keep in touch.

Love, Cindy

MY FIRST JOURNAL ENTRY . . .

Written January 6, 2012 6:06 p.m. by Cindy Marshall

It's amazing to think that less than a month ago I was diagnosed with breast cancer. First there was shock; now there is fear of what is yet to come. The best part is all of my loving family and friends—I can't thank you enough for sending me loving thoughts and prayers! Your strength will help me get through this and I really appreciate it.

I also want to send a HUGE thank you to Team Cindy, who helped me this week. First, my loving boyfriend Craig, who has been by my side since day one and has supported me with tons of love and friendship. We spent the BEST last week of the year in England, his homeland, where he spoiled me with love the entire time. He has been fabulous, and I am SO GRATEFUL to have him in my life! Craig is committed to beating this awful disease with me and ready to partake in the long journey ahead. Thank you, my love!

Secondly, I want to thank Fran Philip, one of my best friends, for spending the week with me. Fran lives in Freeport, Maine, with the most adorable and loving man, George. I am very grateful that she came to help me out, especially given the sudden loss of her father, Stu Dog (my favorite nickname for him), just one month ago. Fran is a ten-year breast cancer survivor, so she knows what to do. She took control and helped me with doctors' visits and creating this site. Stu Dog loved sunflowers and so do I, which is why I have a sunflower theme for the site. I will be dreaming of sunflowers in Provence as I go through my treatments. Thank you, Frannie—you ROCK!

Last, but certainly not least, is Mary Sullivan, an angel on earth, who has been by my side for all the UNC hospital visits so far. Mary is the best friend of Vicky Devlin Jones (Stu Dog's wife and also my very good friend), and she happens to live a few miles from me in Chapel Hill! Mary has been there to hold my hand during the painful needle biopsies (had one today). Additionally, she has been my driver and note taker, along with Fran, so that Craig and I could listen to the doctors.

It's all overwhelming, but the support, strength, and love of Team Cindy has helped a lot! Thank you, Craig, Fran, and Mary!

I ask all of you to pray for me—next week will be another big hurdle. I have my lymph node biopsy surgery on Monday, and we need to pray for negative results—meaning NO cancer in the lymph nodes.

Thank you and I love you all!
Cindy

OVERFLOWING WITH LOVE!!!

Written January 7, 2012 5:51 p.m. by Cindy Marshall

WOW!!! I am SO grateful to have such loving family and friends!! I am now addicted to my sunny CaringBridge website—I can't wait to log on and see what everyone has posted! Thank you for your love, prayers, concern, support, and especially humor. My cup runneth over with LOVE thanks to all of you!

On Monday, December 12th, the Pink Ladies of Vermont sent me this email . . .

Subject: thinking in pink about you, love from the Green (Pink) Mountain State

Hey Cindy Lou Who!!!!!! We are thinking of you while you are going through diagnosis tonight and we're sending vibes to the MRI to get a good outcome. We are gathering at Carol's tonight to wish you well and raise a glass to your recovery, to let you know how much we miss you and think about how to support you. When you get out of the MRI, we hope you will read this and feel our presence embracing you xxxxxxxoooo

Carol, Ellen, Lynn, Andrea, Terry, Ellen, and Annette

The photo was their lovely salute to me.

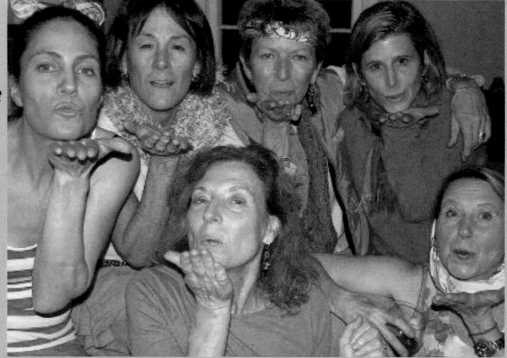

Vermont Pink Ladies—Annette, Carol, Lynn, Ellen, Terry, and Andrea

Thanks, Pink Ladies! I Love You!

ONWARD AND UPWARD

Written January 8, 2012 9:21 p.m. by Cindy Marshall

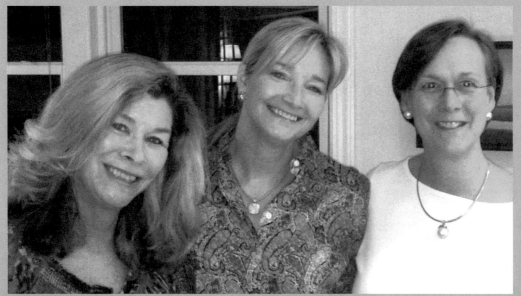

Me with Fran and Mary

Thank you everyone for your kind words, support, love, and prayers. I feel completely blessed and at peace as I prepare for lymph node surgery tomorrow. I do feel the "ring of power" all around me.

I have to share a moving experience I had today with my cousin Davey Diamond. Davey is a minister in Covington, LA, and a miracle man. He prayed with me for thirty minutes today and I felt so peaceful after this. Even Craig said I seem relaxed and serene. Davey shared many healing stories with me and then asked me to repeat after him as we prayed to our beloved Lord. It was very powerful, and I am grateful for my loving cousin Davey!

I am off to bed to get a good night's sleep. I will keep everyone posted about how I am feeling tomorrow. We won't have results until Wednesday. Once I know, you will know. I am learning how to be patient (really, Fran, I am) and to be at peace.

Good night and love to all!
Cindy, aka Whoville

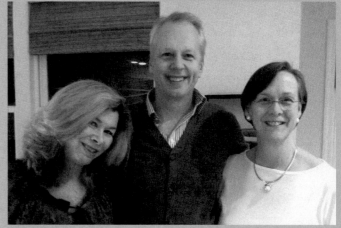

Craig with Fran and Mary

POST SENTINEL NODE SURGERY REPORT

Written January 9, 2012 6:41 p.m. by Craig Waller

Day started at mammography about 8 a.m., where Cindy had four shots of radioactive dye done. Craig was chief hand-holder: great job!! After about thirty minutes, Dr. Amos, the surgeon, came and personally wheeled Cindy (with entourage following) through the maze of corridors from the cancer hospital to the main hospital for surgery. He is just the most fabulous doc and good guy all around. He and Craig even found mutual acquaintances. Plus, he was wearing his lucky Dallas Cowboy socks today!!

Came out of surgery around 11:50. Dr. Amos removed three sentinel nodes about the size of an English pea (very small) and should have the pathology report by Wednesday. He used a little Dermabond on the incision area, so there's no bandage or external stitches. Cindy was in recovery for a while to get the pain under control.

Yes, she did pee blue from the dye, which he used to trace the sentinel node! She's on rest for today and probably tomorrow, will be sore under the armpit area, and is not to lift anything more than ten pounds for two weeks. Cindy will hear from Dr. Amos on the pathology report for today's surgery as well as the right breast core biopsy taken last week.

GREAT NEWS!

Written January 9, 2012 7:13 p.m. by Cindy Marshall

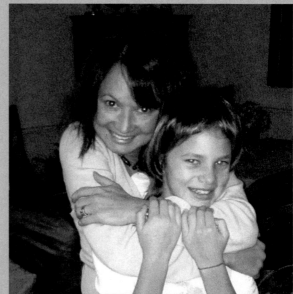

I received a call a little while ago from the geneticist that it is NOT in my genes!! That means I have NO gene mutation—yippee!! The reason this matters is that gene mutation causes higher risk of ovarian cancer and breast cancer returning. I always knew I had magnificent genes!! Thank you, Mom and Dad!!

While I was typing this, my fabulous surgeon, Dr. Amos, called to tell me the right breast biopsy is benign!! Yippee!

Linh and Audrey Calhoun

That means I have double negative so far—just what I wanted!!! The last test result will be from today, and we expect to hear Wednesday. Keep those prayers coming!!

Love to all and thank you Lord!!!

Written January 11, 2012 8:45 a.m. by Cindy Marshall

I didn't think the lymph node surgery would knock me down as hard as it has. I can't use or lift my left arm—it's amazing how much you need both arms! The doctors had me on Percocet Monday, so I didn't have a lot of pain until the middle of the night, so of course I took more. Yesterday I thought I didn't need the meds during the day . . . That was wrong. I pushed too much, and by 3 p.m. I was exhausted and in lots of pain. Good news: the angels on earth came out to help me! Mary came to check on me in the afternoon. She walked Poppy (Craig's dog, who is visiting me), helped me find clothes to wear, and redid my bandage. Then Craig came home to help get me comfortable, take care of me, and share his love. Then Linh Calhoun and her lovely daughter Audrey stopped by with dinner and food for the week! They spoiled us with goodies from Whole Foods. Thank you, Linh and Audrey!! The attached photo is of Linh and Audrey (who happens to be sporting my first wig!)

Thank you everyone for your notes, love, and prayers! You are keeping me going!! It means a lot to me, and I can't wait to check to read more.

I love you all!!

TRIPLE NEGATIVE!!!
Written January 11, 2012 5:42 p.m. by Cindy Marshall

I scored with a triple negative!! Yahoo!! Dr. Amos called me at 4 p.m. today to share the good news—NO cancer in the lymph nodes!!! He told me I am batting 1,000 right now—keep it up!! I am so relieved . . . the prayers worked! Thank you everyone!! Onward and upward—GET ON IT!

ANOTHER TREATMENT TODAY . . .

Written January 12, 2012 9:48 p.m. by Cindy Marshall

YES again, second time this week, I had to get dressed in a "Johnny," have an IV hooked up and get wheeled into surgery! But this time I didn't have general anesthesia, only "conscious sedation." This is when they put you to sleep but for a short period of time and you don't have the terrible side effects of anesthesia. Today was the "port-a-cath" placement that is a small device surgically implanted under the skin, in the upper right chest near the collarbone, that enters a large blood vessel and is used to deliver medicine. All my friends that have had this, or currently have it, say it's SO worth it—you avoid being stuck with a needle every time you have blood drawn or get meds like chemo. So once again I am in pain, but not as bad as Monday AND I am taking my pain medicine.

Mary Sullivan, my angel on earth, was by my side all day. She even helped me pick out some nutrition books from the UNC resource library and shop for groceries. Then I came home to several packages—a care package of food and spices from Kristina and new Tempur-Pedic pillows from Mary Ellen and Mindy. Can't wait to try them out tonight! Then Craig arrived with a warm bag of home-cooked soup and muffins from Bonnie, my former boss at Pace Communications. YUM, YUM!! What a treat!! She even gave me a framed copy of Philippians 4:4–7, which is lovely!

Yesterday, I had several surprises—flowers in the morning from Jaci, my girlfriend at Pace, and her husband Bob, then an afternoon delivery of flowers from my buddies in Maine: Jeff, Kali, Kristen, Brian, Dan, and Dorothy! Thanks!! Then a celebration bouquet from Craig for clean lymph nodes—thanks, my love!! The house smells great, and I am happy.

I also want to thank Mark and Mary for the inspirational books and flowers. Plus, thank you Kris for the chicken soup book! I know I will have lots of time to read and I appreciate the thoughtfulness! And Vicky, my orchid is doing well and keeping me smiling! Thank you everyone for your continued support and love! I can truly say I feel blessed to be alive and have such loving family and friends! You are the best!!

Onward . . . get on it! Love to all,
Cindy

GO PATRIOTS!!!

Written January 14, 2012 8:37 p.m. by Cindy Marshall

Wow!! What a start to the game!! Touchdown in less than two minutes!! I was just starting to write, "Here I sit watching the Patriots . . . ," and they score! I can't thank you enough for the daily updates and messages. You make every day better than the last, and I am so thankful for each and every one of you!

Since I wrote last, I have almost fully recovered from both surgeries this week. YEAH! I am done with meds and now taking Tylenol when needed. I finally took a shower today—after five days it felt GREAT! My port scars are healing well and re-dressed in new bandages. Tom and Zully Blake stopped by with several bags of groceries to make fresh juice concoctions—yippee. They included a great cookbook to help me fight cancer and some awesome tea!

Fran, George, Mary Ann, Hub, John, Nancie, Vicky, Marilyn, Joanne, Ruthie, and the rest of the Sunday River crew—thanks for your messages and keep the slopes ready for me!! See you soon!

Love to all and GO Patriots!! They scored again!!

PREPARING FOR THE HAIRCUT . . .

Written January 15, 2012 9:18 p.m. by Cindy Marshall

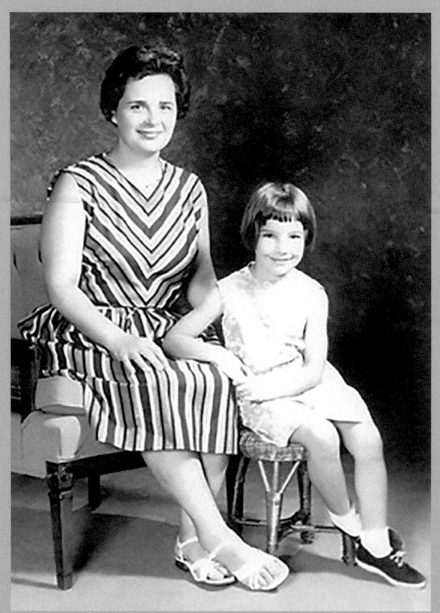

Me with Mom 1969

This is a picture of me with my mother when I was five or six years old—notice the short haircut! This was the last time I had really short hair.

Tomorrow is the big day. I am getting my long Cindy locks cut off, but I know it will grow back (maybe curly this time). I have ordered several wigs and will sport them when needed.

Onward and Get On It!

Love to all,
Cindy, aka Whoville

SPORTING MY NEW SASSY HAIRSTYLE

Written January 16, 2012 1:07 p.m. by Cindy Marshall

I did it!! I got on it and cut my hair!! I only had a few tears in the beginning, but my fabulous hair stylist, Dale, calmed me down with his loving spirit! Here it is—the view from the front! I love it and don't know why I waited so long . . . maybe I was scared, but I feel great, and my hair is healthy! Who knows how long that will last, but I am fine with it now.

We googled "short, sassy haircuts" and found a lot of really fun styles to choose from. We did a combination of a few of them . . . models and actresses combined. Dale—thank you for taking such good care of me!!

Love to all,
Cindy

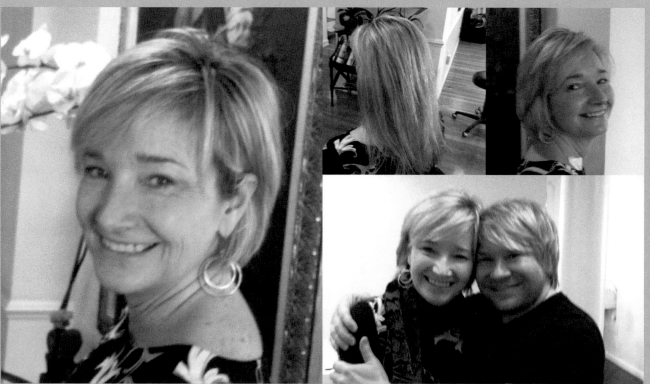

Me with Dale Key, January 2012

THE JOURNEY CONTINUES . . .

Written January 18, 2012 8:11 p.m. by Cindy Marshall

Tomorrow is the big "first day" of chemo—it kind of feels like the first day of school or starting a new job, but then again, I know I can face it. I keep thinking, "It's only eight sessions of chemo; how hard can that be?" Then the realist in me comes out, especially after reading all the literature they gave me, and I know it's the side effects that can be tough. I am holding onto the fact that I WILL KCB (kick cancer's butt), as I am a survivor and always have been. Plus, I have all of you, the best circle of love one could ask for. Thank you!

I chose this picture because it reminds me of a happy moment just short of three weeks ago, toasting to life and love! Onward and upward!

As Stu Dog would say,
"Whoville, GET ON IT"!
I'm on it and I love you all!
Cindy Lou

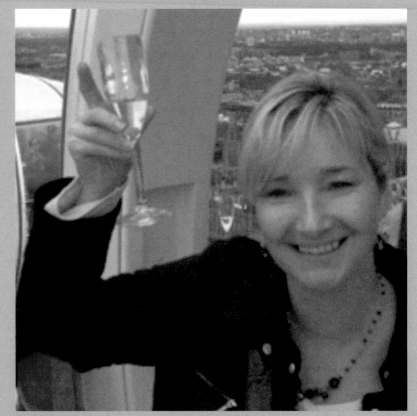

London Eye Toast

FIRST DAY TOWARD SURVIVORSHIP!

Written January 19, 2012 2:03 p.m.
by Cindy Marshall

Team Linh and Mary are here with me. So far, we saw the nurses in oncology that prepared the port with my IV non-coring needle. Then we waited to be seen on the third floor infusion center. They have forty-eight seats to treat patients—holy smoke! Yesterday they had seventy-two patients—what a pervasive disease!! All seats face a window; my window faces the courtyard side and others face the sunny side, but all sides are sunny in my book! Right now, I am having saline solution and premeds (for nausea) infused into my system. This takes an hour, so Mary and Linh went to get us food. I was given several meds orally when we arrived—steroids and anti-nausea. I have about twenty to thirty minutes more before the first chemo drug, Adriamycin, goes in (the red devil, because it's red and kills the cancer!). They flush my port and the second chemo drug, Cytoxan, is infused, which takes an hour. We are thinking closer to 4 p.m. I will be done. Lunch just arrived—Team Cindy is fabulous!

Thank you!!!

I could not have done this without Craig, my lover, and Mary, my angel on earth! They were

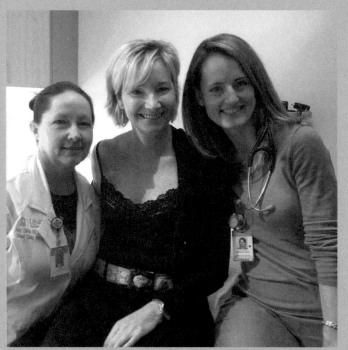
Me with nurses Amy and Anna Kate

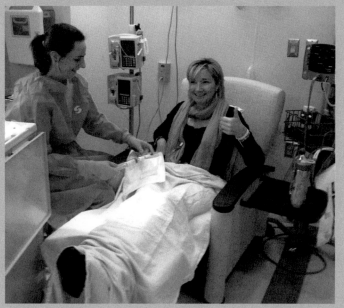
Chemo nurse Kate

beyond supportive and helpful. They made me feel loved, and for that I am so grateful. I think of all the people that don't have anyone to drive them to chemo, to hold their hands, or to be by their side. It makes my heart ache. Here are a few pictures of my first day. I remember chatting with all the nurses, and my chemo nurse Kate, who delivered the red devil, was also a Brit! She was so friendly, and Craig loved chatting with her!

ONE DOWN, SEVEN TO GO . . .

Written January 19, 2012
7:05 p.m. by Cindy Marshall

I'm home and on the couch relaxing. I feel fine right now, but I am sure I will be tired tonight. Long day but first one down and gone! Team Cindy, Linh Calhoun and Mary Sullivan, were fabulous! Thank you ladies, for driving, carrying my big bag, feeding me, making me laugh, and most importantly, loving me!

I was in good hands all day and really like the nurses too. I missed one of Jerome from infusion, but I have seven more chances. My

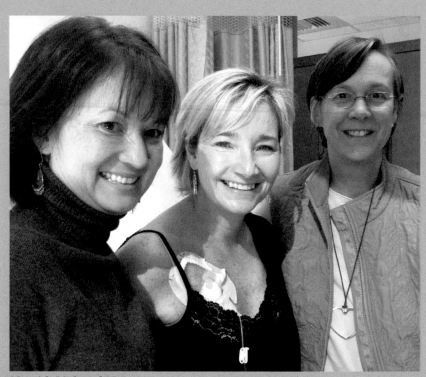

Me with Linh and Mary

chemo nurse, Kate, was a doll—such a sweetheart—and she is British! Things happen for reasons (still not sure why cancer happened to me . . . but not worrying about that now).

Mary Norton, my friend and neighbor, stopped by twice to say hello and give me a goodie bag with chocolates, water, and Tar Heel pins!

My horoscope today was "Concentrating on your commitment to excellence calms your current wanderlust and keeps you on track all day." So true—we stayed focused and on task. There are a lot of emotions that run when anticipating what the day will be like, but now I know; it wasn't too bad. I did get sinus pressure from one of the meds, but that is going away. The side effects are the issue. Sunday (the third day) will be my worst day. Onward to live life to the fullest (sans alcohol)!

To the Sunday River gang, so BUMMED I missed first tracks. I hope you had freshies! LOVED that you skied White Heat in my honor!! Thank you for making this Cindy Day. Now I need to get you "Cindy Lou Who" dolls to wear on your helmets!

OK, enough for now . . .

Thank you all for your continued love, messages, emails, cards, food, support, and prayers and for making me feel so special!

Love to all!
Cindy Lou

THIRD DAY AND SO FAR, SO GOOD!
Written January 22, 2012 12:21 p.m. by Cindy Marshall

Dear Circle of Power and LOVE,
You are the BEST and I am so grateful for all your notes! Thanks everyone for being so good to me!

Quick update . . .

So today is THE third day after chemo and so far, so good. I got twelve hours' sleep last night (needed it, as I didn't sleep Friday night), and I'm feeling fairly good right now. I only ache in my neck, shoulders, and back, almost like I had an intense workout or massage. I will take this over the other potential side effects! The plan for the day is to rest, snuggle up by the fire, and watch the Patriots game later on. GO PATS!!

That's all for now. Happy Sunday!

Love,
Cindy

SECOND TREATMENT TOMORROW

Written February 1, 2012 5:40 p.m. by Cindy Marshall

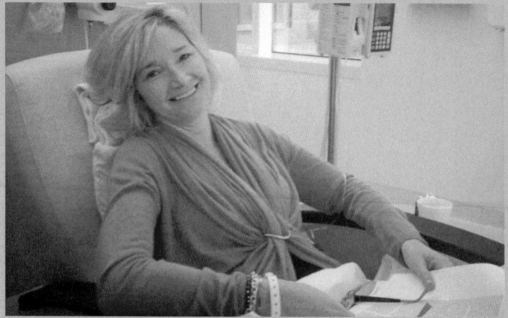

Me doing work during chemo

Hi All,

Thanks for your continued notes and posts. I am feeling so loved and embraced by the circle of power. You are the best! I have another treatment tomorrow, and Craig is my Team Cindy. It starts at 9 a.m. with a blood test, then a visit with the oncology nurse to check in on me, and the last stop will be the infusion room at 11:00. Hopefully, we can be back home by 2:00, but one never knows. I will write again tomorrow with an update to fill you in.

So far all is fine, just a little insomnia. Liz Cook shared her favorite remedy, valerian tea, which I tried last night, and it was great! I didn't like the melatonin—it gave me strange dreams and I felt groggy in the morning. I still have all my hair . . . not sure when that will start to shed, but I am thinking another week. Wig accessories are ready!

GET ON IT!
Love,
Cindy

IT'S STARTING . . .

Written February 4, 2012 4:47 p.m. by Cindy Marshall

Just as my fabulous nurse Anna Kate predicted, my hair is shedding, ugh. She said it would start at the second chemo and I was feeling so proud that no shedding occurred before Thursday. But I knew it was coming, and as I showered Friday night, it was starting to fall out—small bits, not large. So I braved it and went out to visit with a friend I hadn't seen for ten years, Mary Edgerton of Williamstown! The photo is a shot of Mary and me having dinner at the Lantern, my favorite spot in Chapel Hill!

Today, I had a nice day with Craig doing errands and getting ready for SB Sunday! I'm thinking that if my hair continues to shed and my scalp tingles, like Anna Kate said it would, then maybe Super Bowl Sunday is the "shaving day" but still ONE DAY AT A TIME.

Thanks for all your love and support. Your circle of power is amazing and I love you all!

Go PATs—GET ON IT!

Love,
Cindy Lou Who

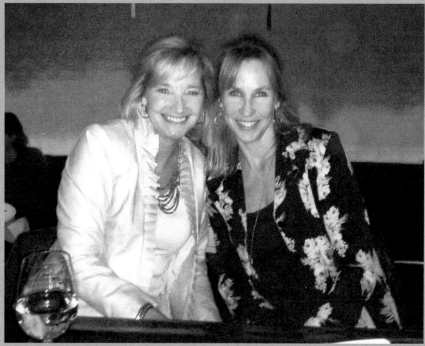

Me with Mary Edgerton

BALD BOMBSHELL

Written February 7, 2012 8:23 p.m. by Cindy Marshall

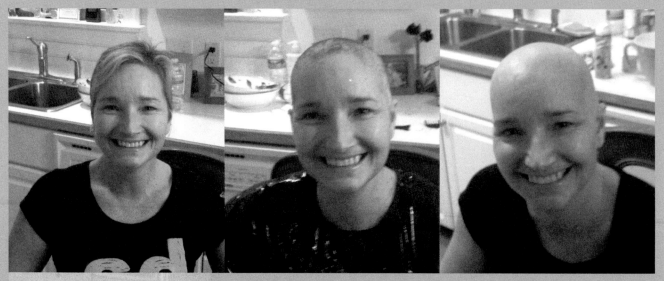

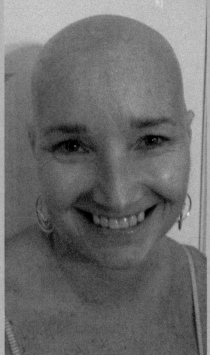

OK Fran, love the name. My HMN has now nicknamed me Hot Bald Bombshell—HBB! Tonight was an experience we will never forget, and Craig was absolutely amazing! Thank you, darling, for your love and gentle touch!!

At first, we were both scared, but then my HMN got the hang of it and zippy do, zippy da, no more hair! We both broke out laughing when his British humor kicked in: "This is like mowing the grass; it's so much fun and you have to be careful not to leave patterns." We used the electric razor to clean my head down to a stubble—about three passes—then the shaving cream and razor came out. It's amazing how much colder it is without hair. I now know what it feels like to be bald, and BALD is BEAUTIFUL!!

Thank you all for your loving support! I feel better now . . . GET ON IT Whoville!

Love and BIG hugs,
Cindy HBB

At some point I had an EKG of my heart, and that was the most magical experience. I know it sounds strange, but while I was going through this emotional and spiritual time, I felt the love of God in the room. I felt light and peace come over me as I listened to my heart beat loud like a washing machine. It made me smile with the wonder of life—how blessed we are to have a heart and to hear it beat. I remember praying that day that I would be able to continue to hear my heartbeat!

MY WORST DAY EVER . . .

Monday, the morning after the Super Bowl, I woke up at Craig's house in a terrible state of mind. I have to say this was my worst day during the chemo! I was told it would be hard to lose my hair, but I didn't realize how hard. As a woman, my hair was so much a part of my femininity and beauty. It frightened me to lose it, and I had no idea how much this would bother me.

We had celebrated the Patriots winning the Super Bowl the night before with Chris, Craig's best friend, and Sophie, Craig's youngest daughter, who were both visiting from London. I was just getting to know both, as my relationship with Craig was still new.

I remember waking that Monday morning; Craig and Chris had already left the house. I had originally planned to work remotely at Craig's house, but I felt awful. There was hair all over my pillow—it was coming out in clumps. I was so shocked, all I could do was cry. I let it happen, and that was a good thing. The sobs were coming so fast, it was one of those uncontrollable cries. All I could think of was sneaking out of the house and driving the hour back to Chapel Hill.

I remember trying to clean up my face, grabbing my travel bag, and opening the bedroom door quietly, trying not to make noise and wake Sophie. As I opened the door, I was greeted by Sophie coming out of her bedroom in her PJs. She saw immediately that I was a mess. She asked if I was OK, which was all it took for me to break down and sob again. I told her about my hair, and she held me with the biggest and tightest hug and said she was sorry. That was a loving and unforgettable moment. It was also a special bonding moment for us.

Work was keeping me going.

Chapter 9

EMBRACING POSITIVITY

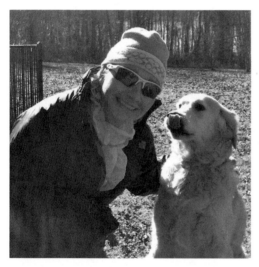

Work was keeping me going as I focused on strategic consulting with Brooks Brothers and helping the sales team respond to marketing database proposals for brands like Estée Lauder, Green Mountain Coffee Roasters, and Gardener's Supply. I was glad to have something to get my mind off treatment and thoughts about survival. I remember feeling sick during this time, but following the doctors' orders was the best thing I could do. I was given so many recommendations of what to do when I felt nauseous, like eating crystallized ginger and drinking tea. This really did help.

UNC Chapel Hill had so much to offer, including nutrition and general exercise classes. I attended many of these classes, and as a result, I made sure I walked every day with Poppy, Craig's dog, who became my "chemo pal." Poppy was truly an angel dog with so much love and companionship. She even liked my cat, Jaguar.

I remember getting tested for vitamin D levels and I was very high, over 70 ng/ml, which was very surprising to the doctors. We realized that it was because I was walking Poppy thirty to sixty minutes daily between 11 a.m. and 2 p.m., the optimal sun times for natural ingestion of vitamin D. Thank you, Poppy girl, for being my chemo pal and buddy!

SNOWING IN ASHEVILLE

Written February 11, 2012 10:49 a.m. by Cindy Marshall

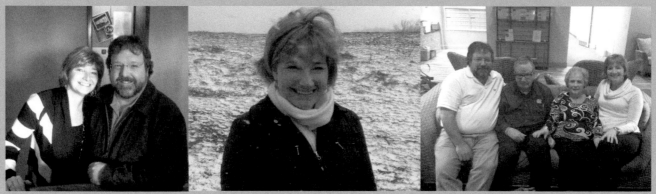

Me with brother Richard and my parents, Ken and Jane

Hi All,

I woke up to snow flurries in Asheville, which was lovely to see. My older brother, Richard, from Miami, came to visit this past Thursday, and we drove up to Asheville on Friday to visit with our parents. I had a little stomach trouble yesterday, but the nausea pills they gave me worked just fine! Today we plan to visit and have a nice lunch out at one of their favorite restaurants, then it's back to Chapel Hill to see Craig and his daughter Sophie.

The attached photo is a picture of me (sporting Meg wig) and Richard at the Top of the Hill, which is one of our famous UNC bars. Richard is a University of Miami alumnus, so he came dressed in Hurricane colors, but I made him take his hat off so he wouldn't get attacked by Tar Heel fans! He gave me two fabulous bracelets and some cards from his family of ladies. One of them has the breast cancer ribbon, and the other has a cross with a lovely saying: "Ask it will be given you, Seek and you will find, Knock and the door will be opened to you." Thank you, Richard, Cindy, Kristen, and Kaitlyn. I love you!

Have a great weekend and thanks for the continued posts!

Love to all!!
Cindy Lou Who

HAPPY VALENTINE'S DAY!!

Written February 14, 2012 6:13 p.m. by Cindy Marshall

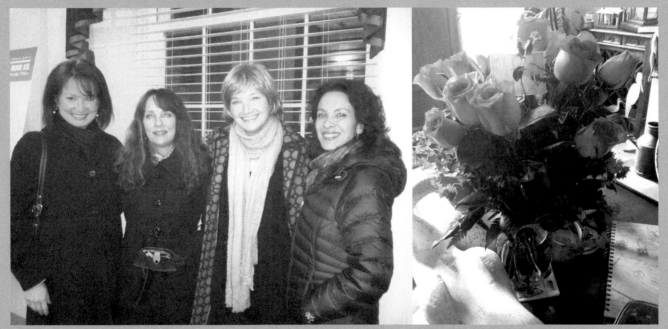

Me with Linh, Melinda, and Zully　　　　　　　　　　　　*Valentine's flowers from my love!*

To My Loved Ones,

Wishing you all a very happy Valentine's Day filled with love and friendship! I had a great day, and I'm now waiting for my adorable man to arrive and head to dinner at Provence, a restaurant in Carrboro that we haven't tried, and I plan to wear my Marseille wig—how appropriate!

The attached photo is a picture of my evening out last night with the girls—Linh Calhoun, Zully Amaya, and Melinda Buleza. We went to dinner at the Top of the Hill and to see Alvin Ailey at the Chapel Hill Performing Arts Center (on UNC campus), which was a real treat!

Love to all and Happy Valentine's to my circle of power!
Cindy

NUMBER THREE DOWN, FIVE MORE TO GO!

Written February 16, 2012 9:11 p.m. by Cindy Marshall

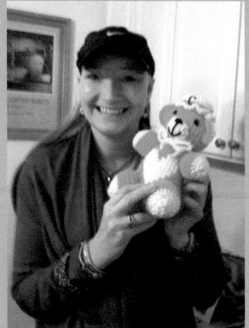

Hi Everyone,

I made it through number three chemo treatment today. It was a long day, as the cancer center was running behind, but there are only five more! Team Cindy consisted of Craig and Mary Sullivan, my angel on earth. I am feeling a bit tired now, so in bed as I write this, but wanted to update everyone. I think I will be extra tired this weekend.

My Aunt Nancy (Dad's sister) and Uncle Clark came to visit last night on their drive south to Florida from Nantucket! We had a nice visit at the house, and then the four of us went to Crooks Corner for a taste of real Southern cooking! It was a special treat to see them, and I thank them both for making the effort!!

Tonight, my good friend who is like a sister to me, Sarah Boudreau, came to visit awhile and we shared a lovely take-out meal from Pazzo's. Sarah is doing a horse show in Raleigh this week, so it was really special for me to see her! For those who don't know Sarah, she is the sister of Fran Philip and lives in Norfolk, VA. Over the past sixteen years, we spent many holidays and lots of weekends together and even lived near each other in Maine. Unfortunately, I didn't manage to get a picture of the two of us. But I did manage to have Sarah take

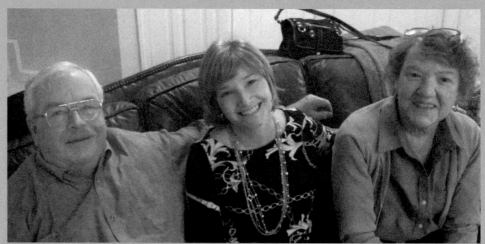

Me with Uncle Clark and Aunt Nancy

a picture of me holding this cute pink cuddle bear made by a special friend of hers. Notice the long hair attached to my baseball cap, just one of my hair accessories . . .

Off to sleep, tired but doing OK. GET ON IT!

Love to all,
Cindy Lou Who

HAPPY PRESIDENT'S DAY

Written February 20, 2012 7:53 p.m. by Cindy Marshall

Hi Everyone,
I started my day by attending a "Look Good Feel Better" class at the UNC Cancer Center. This is a free session teaching cancer patients how to take care of their skin while undergoing chemo treatments. We received a bag full of beauty products, from makeup to facial cleansers and creams, probably a $150 value! I learned a lot and met some other women dealing with similar issues. The hard part was meeting ladies that have lung cancer, brain tumors, and ovarian cancer with little time left. I have to say this was a big moment for me—they were so upbeat and positive about life, never quitting. It gave me renewed strength, but it made me sad for them. It also made me grateful for not having to deal with something worse, like a brain tumor. There is light at the end of the tunnel, and I am thankful daily for the life I have and for all of you!!

My good friend Diane Scott volunteers in Boston to teach this class so I was feeling very close to her today! I learned how to make a T-shirt turban—they even used my Hot Bald Bombshell (HBB) as the model to show the class! What a hoot! I also learned how to tie a scarf, add pins and flowers to hats, and wash a wig. We discussed the hygiene aspect of everything we do—always wash your hands, use gloves to clean, be very careful with manis and pedis (make sure their products are sanitized), and make sure you always use sunscreen, even when wearing a wig. I also learned a few new makeup tips! So all in all, it was a great class and good for me to meet some other patients. I felt good and looked better afterward; I even ran into my nurse, Amy, in the hall, and she told me how great I looked!

Afterward, I visited briefly with my AOE, Mary Sullivan, at her home in Fearrington Village. Her close friend Nita knitted me a beautiful purple "treatment shawl full of positive energy," which blew me away! I have only met Nita once, but she is one of Mary's closest friends and wanted to do something for me. I am so blessed.

I made it through another post-chemo weekend and did fairly well. I do have to say it's like clockwork—by 9 p.m. Saturday night, I hit a wall with fatigue and full-body aches. Easy to fix with my heating pad and HMN! I rested and got the sleep I needed this weekend, so I am feeling good today but taking it one day at a time.

Thank you everyone for your continued love, prayers, support, and positive mojo!! YOU ROCK!

GET ON IT—only five more to go!
Love,
Cindy Lou

ANGELICA GOES TO THE MOVIES
Written February 25, 2012 6:04 p.m. by Cindy Marshall

Hi All,
It's been a while since I posted, partly because I had a lot of fatigue this week. Monday was a good energy day, but Tuesday and Wednesday were very weak energy days. I took it easy, did my work—which helps me get my mind off things—and by Thursday I was feeling somewhat normal again. I also had more nausea feelings this time so stayed on the pills longer than round two (seven days vs. five days). My good friend Kim Woodhouse told me it was best to stay ahead of it, so I did. She also helped me a lot this week when I was low and had no energy, as she has been through this before. Thank you, Kimmy!!

Thursday night, I went to a UNC class on nutrition for preventing cancer, which was taught by two fabulous young UNC oncology nutritionists. I am so glad I went. There were only ten people in the class, so we were able to interact and participate. I ran into one of the ladies I met on Monday at the Look Good Feel Better class, and she gave me a big hug. I learned that we should all have five servings of cruciferous vegetables weekly; these are from the mustard family, and they include broccoli, brussels sprouts, cabbage, kale, mustard greens, and cauliflower. OK, time to start eating more veggies. Craig and I love asparagus, so we have that often, which is still good, but it's time to add some more to our diets. They also discussed resveratrol, which comes from red grapes (yes, red wine is good), dark chocolate, and peanuts!! They said we need to make this part of our daily diet; that doesn't mean drink tons of red wine, but a glass or two is good for you. One great idea that was shared was to freeze red grapes and eat them like popsicles—yum! We make a kale and berry salad along with a lentil hummus; both were excellent. I got plenty of literature and a few new recipes. Well worth the time!

Friday night, Craig and I went to see The Artist, and tonight we are off to see Hugo in 3D! We are trying to see as many Oscar movies as possible to be fully up to speed for tomorrow night. So the picture attached

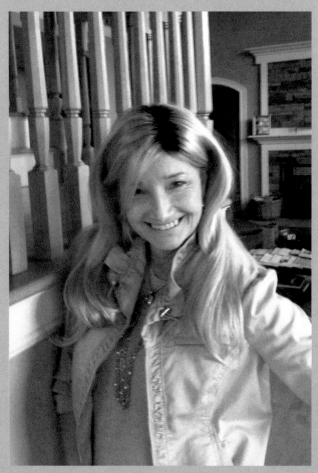

is Cindy sporting the Angelica wig—long blonde bombshell. It's almost a Pamela Anderson or Elle McPherson look but hey, why not have fun with it!

I also received a fabulous package of goodies from my "Big Sishta" Joan Litle. Joan is a longtime industry friend, and we have always said we were sisters! She sent me a great bear that whistles at you. I love him. You press his belly, and he whistles away! She sent me a bottle of Evian water spray for the hot flashes, socks, a lip bracelet, and a butterfly bracelet. All very nice and full of love. Thanks, Joan. You are the BEST and I love you!

Then Diane Scott, my beauty friend, send me a great package of facial beauty products designed specifically for chemo treatment. I started using them and really like them! Thank you, Diane!! I love you!

So Angelica is signing off . . . heading to the movies! I love you all and thanks for your continued support!! Cindy

50% COMPLETE TOMORROW!!

Written February 29, 2012 6:20 p.m. by Cindy Marshall

YIPPEE! I am really excited to think that by this time tomorrow night, I will be officially 50% complete with chemo treatments! Yeah!! I had more fatigue this time, but I guess it's expected when my body is being fed poison to kill cancer. I am so grateful for all of you. I check the site several times a day to see what's new and who left me messages. Thank you for my "ring of power." You are definitely helping me get through this journey!!

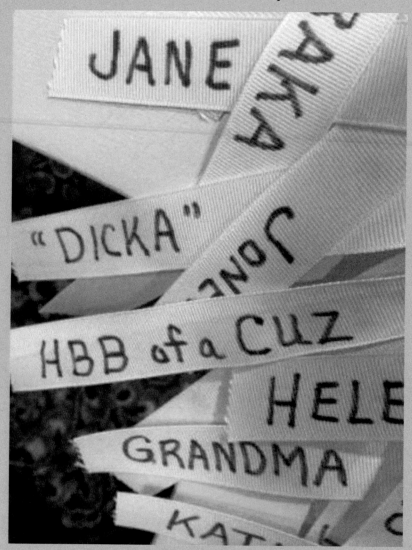

The attached photo is from my cousin Tally, who lives in Albany during the warmer seasons and Florida during the colder months. She was getting ready for a Cure event in Florida, where they made a big pink ribbon filled with little pink ribbons for their loved ones. Tally added a ribbon for me titled "HBB of a Cuz." I love it and I love you Tally!!

When I got home, a package arrived from Fran—a box full of seven bangle bracelets from Alex and Ani. Her note said they are for Happy Spring, Happy St. Patrick's Day, and Happy halfway through chemo. One has a Young and Strong charm, one has a "C" charm, and one has an "everything happens for a reason" charm. Twenty percent of the proceeds are donated to a cancer center! The box contained several cards that explain what these symbols mean—very cool!! Thank you, Fran. I love them and I love you!

Onward and upward . . . tomorrow the chemo van, a luxury Lexus driven by AOE Mary Sullivan, will pick me up at 8:30 to start another round. Mary has been my saint. I am so grateful for her. Thank you, Mary!! I will take my new chemo throw from Nita to stay warm.

Much love to all and GET ON IT!
Cindy, aka HBB Whoville

I pulled on my big girl panties
and told myself I CAN do this,
and I WILL do this. I can lead the
NEMOA conference as president.

Chapter 10

WHO DO I WANT TO BE TODAY?

March began. I was not sure how I was supposed to feel, but I remember feeling nervous, anxious, and scared. First, I was nervous because I was now the president of a very important organization in the multichannel retail world, NEMOA (National Etailing and Mailing Organization of America), that has been around since 1947 and was led by many industry experts and icons. *How was I going to be able to compete with them? How could I stand up to them?* I was going through cancer and chemo. I had no hair. I was on lots of medications. I was about to meet the postmaster general of the United States! I can't handle this, I thought. Second, I was anxious about getting re-imaged to see if the chemo was working. And third, I was scared to travel and be exposed to others while on chemo.

I pulled on my big girl panties and told myself I CAN do this and I WILL do this. I can be the president of NEMOA and lead the annual conference!

While at the board meeting the day before the conference, I decided I would include my fabulous board members and industry friends in the decision of what wig to wear to meet the postmaster general. At the end of our board meeting, I whipped off my "short and sassy" wig and asked the team, "What wig should I wear tomorrow to meet the postmaster general?" At first, they were all shocked to see my bald head, but when they realized I was laughing, they begin to laugh and relax. I brought them into my world. I let down my walls and became vulnerable for them. I tried on two other wigs, and we all decided as a team which one to wear! It was such a memorable moment for me. Not only did we become closer as a board, but they also accepted me for me, not for my hair or my clothes or my position. It was NOT about the hair! I was thrilled to have help, and yes, I asked for it, which was very unlike pre-cancer Cindy.

RENEWED ENERGY!

Written March 8, 2012 9:22 p.m. by Cindy Marshall

I'm on the back end stretch and made it through chemo number four! The worst days for me have been Sunday, Monday, and Tuesday afterward—fatigue, aches, and sick tummy. I stayed ahead of the nausea pills this time, which helped. I rested when I needed to and went to bed early every night, especially Sunday, when I was really low.

I got this sense of renewed energy mid-week—not sure why, but maybe it's because I am past number four, which my oncologist told me was the worst one. I went to Pilates and yoga classes this week, plus I rode my trainer and took several long walks at lunchtime (can't beat the 70+ weather). The exercise and stretching felt good, because I haven't had much energy the past month. I am now focused on body, mind, and spirit, and it feels terrific!

I saw the plastic surgeon Monday, and that was tough. There was a lot to think about and many decisions to be made, but now I feel better about it. I know that God will lead me to the right decision and I don't need to rush it.

I also received several new packages this week; all of you continue to amaze me with your support! Sheila Sullivan sent me a great book that I can't put down, *The Happiness Project.* Leann Griesinger sent me some fabulous PJs from Soma that help absorb the hot flash sweats. They are perfect. Andrea Syverson sent me a gift certificate a few weeks ago to White House Black Market, one of my favorite stores! So I went shopping last Saturday to redeem it; they have a great new spring line! AND Andrea sent me a lovely wall hanging from Colorado this week that says, "Be brave." So thoughtful of you, Andrea. Thank you!

I'm looking forward to a nice spring weekend in Chapel Hill with my HMN. Onward and GET ON IT! So excited to have some energy back. Pray that it stays!!

Love to all and thanks again for your continued support!!
Cindy

HAPPY DAYLIGHT SAVINGS

Written March 12, 2012 8:55 p.m. by Cindy Marshall

Happy Early Spring to Everyone!
I am so happy to have extra daylight time! Yippee! This means evening walks and bike rides!

I am taking my first trip tomorrow since December. Off to Boston for the NEMOA Spring 2012 directXchange conference. I am excited to travel, and I will try to be really careful with germs. NEMOA is a sixty-five-year-old organization that focuses on education and networking within the direct marketing industry, specifically catalogers and retailers. I have been on the board for about ten years and have attended their events for twenty-five years. On Thursday, I will be elected as president of the organization!! I'm very excited about this, and it's a huge honor to me. Everyone at NEMOA has been extremely supportive of my situation as they know I will be fine, just like I do! Wish me luck!

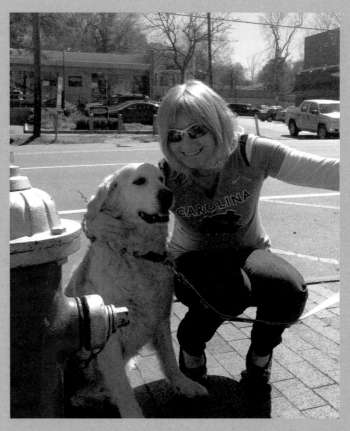

The photo is of me and Poppy on Saturday in downtown Chapel Hill. Craig and I started our day off with a nice bike ride, and then we met Mary and Ed, who live next door, at the Dead Mule pub in Chapel Hill to watch the UNC Tar Heels beat NC State!! It was a close game but a good one! Of course, I was wearing my new Tar Heel shirt that Richard, my brother, gave me for my birthday. Perfect day!

I am feeling great today. I went to an evening yoga class, which is really helping me breathe and open up the tight muscles. Onward and upward—GET ON IT!

Love to all!
Cindy

PS: The wig (Utopia) is my favorite right now.

63% DONE!!

Written March 17, 2012 7:57 p.m. by Cindy Marshall

Hi Everyone,

Yesterday was my fifth treatment—only three more to go! It was a very long day. I started at 10 a.m. and got home at 8 p.m. Mammo, ultrasound, lab work (blood drawn), met with oncologist, four and a half hours in the infusion chair, and finally an MRI at the end of the day. Team Cindy consisted of Craig and Mary. They were great; Craig made a special trip to get us BLTs from Merritt's for lunch. YUM!

I started a new drug called Taxol, and it was taxing. They gave me a large dose of Benadryl as a premed, which completely knocked me out. The good news of the day is that the ultrasound showed that my tumor shrunk from 2.2 cm to 1.5 cm! Great news! Now we have to wait to see what the MRI tells us, because half of my mass can only be seen via MRI. That will be Tuesday, when I meet with Dr. Amos, my breast surgeon.

I had a great week with lots of energy, which helped me get through the NEMOA spring conference event. I am happy to say that I was elected as the president of this fabulous organization; I am thrilled! Lots of work ahead of us over the two-year term but we have a great board, so it will be a team effort!

I am feeling good today. Doctors said it will be seventy-two hours after treatment that I may be sore with body aches. Good news is that there is no nausea with this drug and less fatigue. So, one day at a time I continue. All will be fine.

Thank you everyone for your love and support! I am grateful for my circle of power and love! Onward as we GET ON IT!

Happy St. Patrick's Day!
Much love,
Cindy aka HBB

HAPPY SPRING!
Written March 22, 2012 11:05 p.m. by Cindy Marshall

Many have asked about my recent tests. I had a mammo and an ultrasound last Friday, which showed my tumors shrunk! I also had an MRI, but results didn't come back until Wednesday. My breast surgeon called me at home last night to tell me the MRI mass has gone down as well! He compared them side by side, and the area has reduced, but it's not a concentrated area like a tumor—it's more spread out—so he can't compare size (scattered cancer cells). The good news is that my body is doing what it's supposed to do: it's reacting to the chemo and killing the cancer. Yeah! This is what they want; they don't want the cancer growing and mine is not. So, your prayers and circle of love are working. Thanks, everyone!!

I am having a tougher time with this chemo drug (body aches and fatigue) but taking it one day at a time. Every day I get stronger!

Wishing you all a happy weekend!!

GET ON IT!
Love,
Cindy

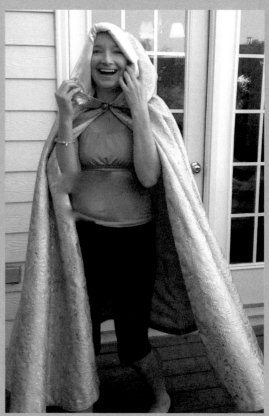

PINK LADIES OF VERMONT SURPRISE ME!
Written March 28, 2012 9:43 p.m. by Cindy Marshall

Hi All,
Today, I picked Andrea Diehl up at the airport, who is one of my close girlfriends from Vermont (one of the cycling babes). She came down to be with me for chemo number six tomorrow. We had a great afternoon touring Chapel Hill and even went for a bike ride on cruisers around the Southern Village neighborhood.

The big surprise was a handmade gift from the girls in Vermont, aka the PINK LADIES, a silk CAPE to wear to chemo!! It is absolutely beautiful and very well made by Terry Findeisen and signed by all the pink ladies:

> *We love you, Cindy Lou, Momma Carol*
> *You're CAPEable of anything! Lynn*
> *For Cindy Lou Who! March 26, 2012, Our Super Girl! XO Terry!*
> ****Fly Cindy FLY!! Annette****
> *Go WONDERful Woman! XO Andrea*
> *Always keep something beautiful in your mind-XOX. Ellen*

WOW! I'm overwhelmed by love. Thank you, ladies!!
Off to number six tomorrow with Team Cindy, Mary and Andrea!
GET ON IT

ONLY TWO LEFT—YIPPEE!
Written March 29, 2012 9:47 p.m. by Cindy Marshall

Today was a good chemo day. I had Team Cindy, consisting of Mary Sullivan (AOE), Andrea Diehl (great girlfriend from Vermont), and my new princess "SUPER girl" cape from the Vermont Pink Ladies! I wore the cape all day, and everyone went nuts—I was stopped frequently and people wanted to read the notes on the bottom. It was lots of fun.

We were serenaded by a talented guitarist, Al, as we entered the infusion room (where chemo is given), and he sang "Edelweiss" to me!!! It was so moving! I got teary at the end as it reminded me of our fabulous Stu Jones's seventy-fifth birthday party at Sunday River with all the gang (five years ago). Some guests dressed up as Sound of Music characters (Marilyn was the Abbess, and Joann wore lederhosen, to name

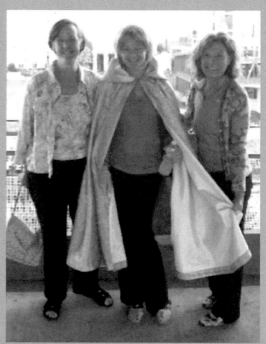

Me with Mary and Andrea

a few) and we sang songs from the movie in honor of Stu. Of course, "Edelweiss" was one of our favorites. Al also sang "Do-Re-Mi" in Hawaiian! What a hoot, though much harder for us to follow.

I made it through treatment fairly well. I didn't have strange effects from the Benadryl like last time, but that is because my dosage was less, and it was taken orally versus through IV. I had a little nap while the ladies went to pick up BLTs for lunch. YUM! I am now resting with Andrea and watching Season 2 of *Downton Abbey,* which I recorded. I am tired . . .

Much love to all and thanks again for all the great posts! GET ON IT and enjoy every NEW day; they are precious.

XOXO
Cindy Lou Who, CAPEable of kicking cancer in the butt!

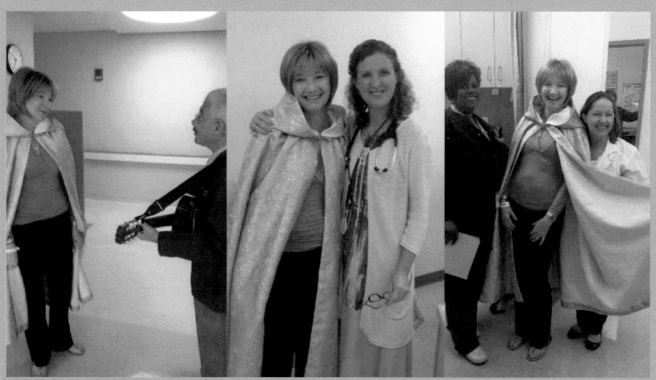

Me with nurses Anna Kate and Amy

April was a tough month. It was also a very life-altering month.

Chapter 11

. . . BY THE WAY, YOU'RE FIRED!

April was a tough month. I remember being up and down all the time. It was also a very life-altering month. My position at Merkle was eliminated. Yes, I was let go and lost my job during my chemo. I found out that the chemo was working, and my tumors were reduced by half! I had to travel and lead my first NEMOA board meeting as president. I had a visit from one of my best friends, Andrea, who lived in Vermont. I also had an interview with senior executives at National Geographic about a potential project.

How do you remain positive and upbeat when your body is on the last month of four months of chemo? Chemo is cumulative. The fatigue was real. It was so hard. I can't even explain how painful it felt when I was alone at night. I cried a lot, but I also tried to stay focused on work to take my mind off things, and I also gave in to bad days—just let it be and go through it. Daria also told me to "go THROUGH it." That helped. It takes more energy to fight it. I became extremely grateful for having my pal Jaguar by my side. He snuggled with me and adored me with unconditional love. I also received so much love from Craig and his dog, Poppy. They were always with me and comforting me as needed. So grateful!

Easter was also in April, and I felt a renewed sense of peace. I believed I would beat this terrible cancer and be OK. One of the things I wanted to do was to give back, so I did it by handing out candy to all the other cancer patients going through treatment on my off-treatment week. I wore my cape, dressed in white, no wig, and a big smile. It was so gratifying. I loved giving others hope, and seeing their smiles filled my heart with love—just like the Grinch's heart expanded, so did mine.

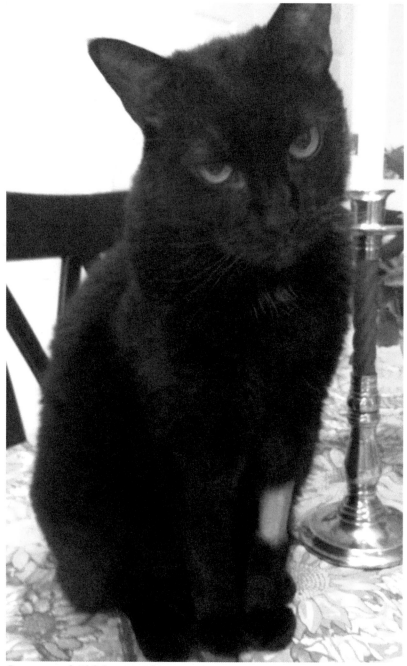

Jaguar, my faithful companion

When I was let go from my job, I let go of my fears and took a deep breath to carry on. It was a blessing in disguise. I had negotiated a severance package when I took the position. This was a message from God to slow down, take care of Cindy, and focus on healing! I received several strong messages from my angels in heaven to take care of me. So that's what I did!

MORE ANGELS ON EARTH

Written April 3, 2012 7:49 p.m. by Cindy Marshall

I had a tough weekend with lots of body aches and no energy. I am so thankful to both Andrea Diehl and Craig, my HMN, for taking such good care of me. I also have to say that I am extremely grateful for Andrea's visit this past week! She is definitely another angel on earth (AOE). She cooked amazing meals for all three of us, cleaned the house, pampered me with my heating pad when needed, walked Poppy (Craig's dog), and cleaned up after herself (sheets, towels, trash, etc.). Andrea was totally fine when I had no energy and couldn't do a thing. She would take a bike out to ride the neighborhood and report back on her visits. Thank you SO MUCH Andrea for being here!! And thank you Mary, AOE, for driving Andrea to the airport on Monday!

The post picture is our night out in Chapel Hill last Friday. I was feeling OK then, so we both dressed up and accompanied Craig to downtown Chapel Hill. It was my first outing in public as HBB—totally bald—and I didn't get any strange looks, so now I am feeling more comfortable going out without my hair accessories! One step at a time, right?!

I also have to send BIG thanks to Laura Hnatow for sending me a lovely white cotton pajama set from Cuddledown. It's so awesome and even buttons down the front, which I will need after surgery. Laura also posted on her Facebook that she decided to ride the Dempsey Challenge, which is a cancer fundraiser that takes place in Maine every October, in my honor!! WOW—very cool. For those who don't know, Laura and I worked together at L.L.Bean on the Freeport Studio business, and now she leads ecommerce at Cuddledown. Laura and I have become great friends over the years, and I am grateful to have her in my life. Please keep her in your prayers today, because she had a spinal tap at Maine Med—one of the tests they are doing to find a CSF leak. Sending you lots of MOJO Laura!!

I am starting to feel better today. Yippee—less aches and pains. Thank you everyone for your continued love and support!!

GET ON IT!!
Love and hugs to all,
Cindy

Me with Andrea

HAPPY EASTER!

Written April 7, 2012 5:04 p.m. by Cindy Marshall

I wanted to wish you all a very happy Easter weekend. I am spending the weekend with Craig in Asheville, NC, visiting my parents. The weather has been lovely—crisp in the morning and 70° in the afternoon with bright blue skies.

My father loves to tell jokes, so here is an Easter joke from Ken, my dad. "What do you call six bunnies moving backward? A receding hare line!" HA! HA!

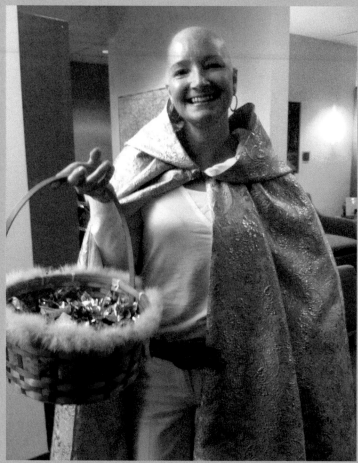

Me handing out candy to cancer patients on Easter

I also want to share a few ups and downs of my week. I keep thinking that life is like a roller coaster ride. I loved going to Kings Dominion as a kid and riding the highest roller coasters with my brothers and friends. I hated it when we were down in the valley. I loved the climb up, and riding over the hill was so exhilarating. Maybe this is why I like skiing so much!

Thursday was my UP ride for the week. I dressed up in all white, put on my CAPE, and went to UNC to hand out Easter candy to all the nurses, doctors, and chemo patients. It was such a hoot!! It made me so happy to see others happy—everyone loved it, and many patients asked for two pieces of candy. I handed out close to a hundred pieces! The photo attached is me as the CAPE-able bunny with PINK basket of candy. I felt so good giving back to all. I am still on an UP ride being here in Asheville with Craig and my parents!

Wednesday was the DOWN part of the week. The strategic consulting team I was part of at work was eliminated and we were all laid off. So I lost my job, which is not good timing, but I am a survivor and will carry on. I will focus on my health over the next few months and start to think about what to do next. One day at a time.

Easter is a sign of new beginnings, so to all a Happy Easter!
MUCH Love,
Cindy
GET ON IT!

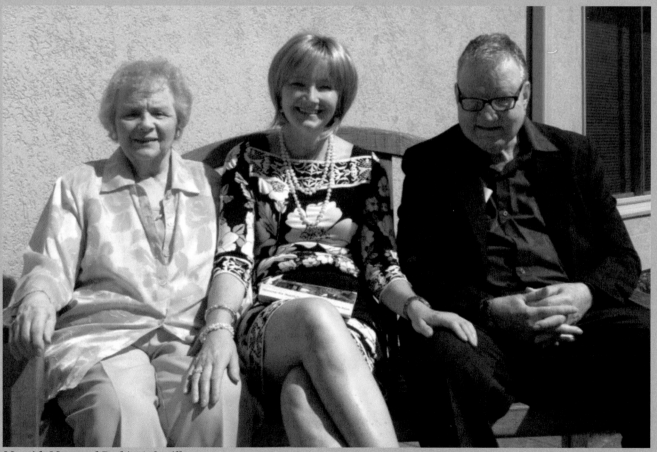

Me with Mom and Dad in Asheville

ONLY ONE CHEMO LEFT—YAHOO!

Written April 13, 2012 1:43 p.m. by Cindy Marshall

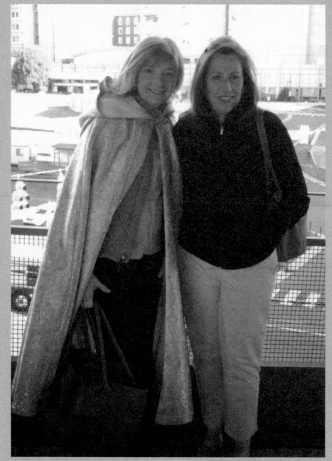

Me with Kim Woodhouse

Yesterday was my seventh chemo, and I feel so good to be almost done!! Team Cindy consisted of Mary Sullivan (AOE), my good friend Kim Woodhouse (visiting from Newport), and Craig, my HMN! We were on time most of the day and had good reports from my oncology nurse Anna Kate. I was told that I am their poster child—always smiling and so positive! I get it from all your support. Thanks! Even the nurse who checks me in to do my vitals says she loves to see me—it's refreshing because I am a "glow of light" and always happy. She said so many people come in so depressed that it makes her day to see me. WOW, that was big. I feel honored. I must have gotten this from my family with great genes that always taught me to see life with a "glass-half-full mentality."

Craig showed up from NYC and brought us some fabulous macarons from Macaron Cafe; they were the best we had ever had!! He even went to Merritt's for lunch—we all had their famous BLTs—the best around. It's becoming our chemo lunch! Thanks sweetie!

The picture is Kim with me in my cape outside of the hospital on our way into treatment number seven at 8:45 a.m. Thank you, Kimmy, for being here. It means so much and it's just like having a sister! I love you!

Kim brought me a very special gift. When Kim was going through lung cancer five years ago, her girlfriends got together and organized a weekly delivery of Hermes scarves with a poem during her chemo. Some were new and some were used, but all were very special. She picked one to pass on to me, which is absolutely beautiful—blue and yellow (my favorite colors) with a horse theme! THANK YOU, Kimmy; you made me cry. It's very special, and I will take good care of it!

I continue to be overwhelmed by the love and support of everyone. Life is beautiful, and you all ROCK!! Thanks for sending me strength, mojo, prayers, and love!

Happy weekend to all!
Love,
Cindy
GET ON IT

WEEK SIXTEEN IS HERE!
Written April 23, 2012 10:13 a.m. by Cindy Marshall

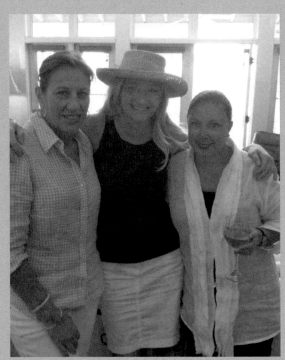
Me with Kim and Karen

WOW, I can't believe that my last week of chemo is here! When I started on January 19, I thought that sixteen weeks was an eternity, and it seemed like the end would never get here. But now it's here, and I feel strong today! My last chemo will be Friday, April 27! I can't thank you enough for all your love, prayers, support, and mojo along the way. I am almost done with one stage of the journey, then it's time to relax before I tackle the surgery stage.

I am writing TWO posts because I have so much to share from the past week.

Last time I wrote, I told you about my friend Kim Woodhouse, who was visiting for chemo number seven. Well, let me tell you she is truly an ANGEL on earth! She pampered me, cooked for me, and helped me around the house. We actually redecorated my downstairs on Friday, April 13. Kim has a spectacular decorating eye, having been in retail for many years. She is a stylist at heart and clearly knows what works and doesn't. She even polished all my silver and cleaned my crystal, then redecorated my dining room hutch and sideboard!! I absolutely LOVE it, and it makes me smile every time I look around, because I think of Kimmy.

Kim drove us to Charleston on Sunday the 15th because she needed to be there for a sailing regatta. We stayed in Charleston Place Sunday night after a nice afternoon walking around old town and having dinner. I joined Kim and her friends at a lovely beach house on Sullivan's Island until Wednesday. The house was just remodeled and right on the water—magnificent views and very peaceful. It was a perfect place for me to rest and listen to the waves crashing! I even made some new girlfriends—Deneen Demourkas, Bunny Wayt, and Jocelyn Thompson—whom I am look forward to getting to know better.

On Tuesday night, we visited with good friends Marc and Karen Hollerbach from Grosse Pointe, MI. It was so fun to see them and reconnect! The attached picture is Kim, Cindy (in Pam Anderson wig), and Karen. What fun!

In the meantime, I received a care package from one of my best friends, Daria, with Irish chocolate (yum— my fav) and a friendship book with daily quotes. Thanks, Daria. I love you!

Thank you for your continued love!
Onward . . .
Love,
Cindy

LOBSTER LOVE

Written April 23, 2012 10:31 a.m. by Cindy Marshall

I had a wonderful visit with my girlfriend Jill Gravel from Portland, ME, on Saturday, April 21. Jill was here visiting her daughter Amy, who goes to High Point University, so we met at the Proximity Hotel Print Works Bistro for lunch. Jill was one of the Freeport Studio team at L.L.Bean and still works at L.L.Bean in women's. She is a fabulous lady with a big heart and a great sense of humor; I really enjoyed spending some quality time with her. Amy, Jill's daughter, was one of our models for Freeport Studio, and now she is in college!! I also saw pictures of David, her fifteen-year-old, who was just a toddler when we worked together. Time flies . . .

Jill brought me a gift from Maine—an Alex and Ani bracelet with a lobster on it. This is what the card says:

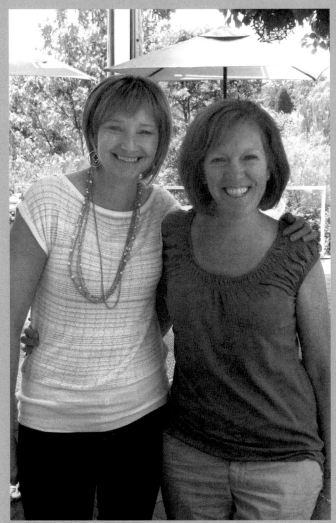
Me with Jill Gravel

Lobster
Cycles|Regeneration|Protection

The lobster is associated with the cycles of the moon and ebb and flow of the tide. Lobsters cast off their shells for new ones. Guided by intuition, they know how to camouflage themselves when in danger. Wear the lobster and learn how to let go of the past, go with the flow, and protect yourself through life's changes.

This means a lot to me! I will wear my lobster bracelet with the rest of the Alex and Ani bracelets from Fran this Friday for my last day of chemo; that way all my Maine friends will be with me!

GET ON IT!
Love,
Cindy

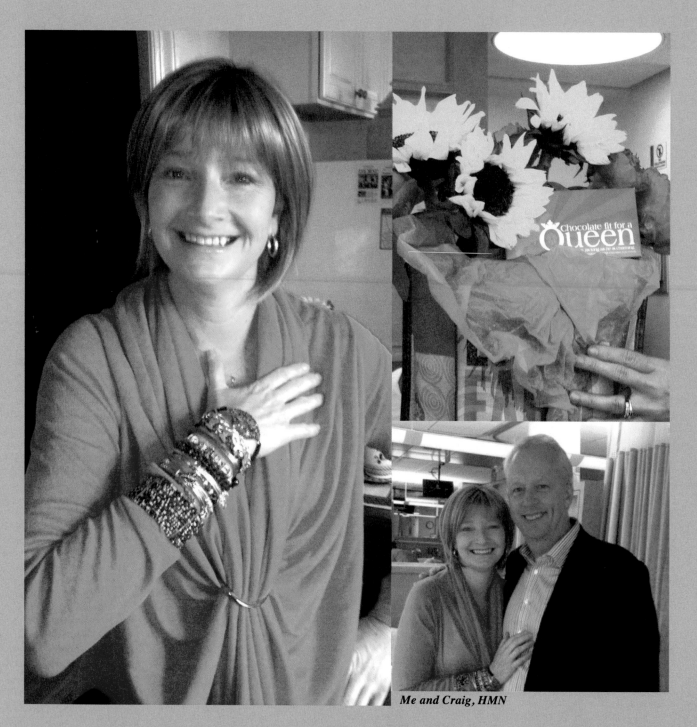

Me and Craig, HMN

I'M DONE WITH CHEMO!!!

Written April 29, 2012 1:28 p.m. by Cindy Marshall

Yippee!!! I can't tell you how relieved I am to be done with this part of the journey! I became impatient five minutes before we were done—I just wanted out of the hospital—but then the nurses delivered my "purple heart award" for completing chemo. It was such a moving experience. They sang "For She's a Jolly Good Fellow" and "Don't Come Back, Jack." Mary Sullivan, my AOE, wore her wings the entire day!!! What a hoot!! Mary, you have been such a pillar of strength for me. Thank you for all you have done!!!

This week was wonderful—so much happened. First, I saw Joan and Tim Litle and Leann and Paul Griesinger Monday night. We started with a visit at Joan and Tim's, then the four of them treated me to dinner in Concord. Then I was off to a NEMOA board meeting, the first one I led as president, which went well. We had a lot of work to do and managed to accomplish most of it!

I spent Tuesday afternoon with Joan, my big sishta, having tea and catching up on life. It was such a special treat to have this time together. Tuesday night was spent with my very good friends Stefanie and Rob Jandl and their daughter Elise (and new Maine Coon cat, Pooky). We had such a great time. Wednesday morning, I had a little more time to spend with Stefanie before I caught my flight home.

Thursday was a day of rest and regrouping before final chemo on Friday. GOOD news: the tumor mass that can be seen via ultrasound shrunk again (from 1.5 cm midway to 0.9 cm)!! The doctors said I responded well to chemo, and they were very proud of me. Yippee!! Tom and Zully Blake brought

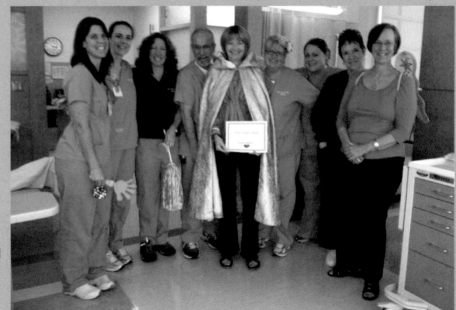

Me with Mary and UNC nurses for last chemo

me dinner on Friday night (yummy Indian from Mint) and a beautiful plant. So special. Thank you both; it meant a lot to me!!!

It will take two full weeks to get the chemo out of my system. I am not taking the white blood cell booster shot this time, so that means less body aches, but I still expect the early part of this week to be tough. My hair will start to grow in three to four weeks, and the doctors said it would be baby fine, brand-new fuzz! Imagine being able to start over with hair. Can't wait to see what color it will be and if it will be straight or curly. Another part of the journey . . .

Michelle Farabaugh, my good friend and former colleague, sent me a lovely Tiffany heart necklace symbolizing new beginnings, strength, and love. She has one as well and wears it in my honor to send me strength!! Carol Freden, who is like a mom to me, sent me handmade pink knitted socks to keep me warm!! They are full of her love and hugs, and I can feel them. Caroline Thompson sent me a necklace with her favorite bible verse, Jeremiah 29:11— *"For I know the plans I have for you"* declares the Lord, *"plans to prosper you and not to harm you, plans to give you hope and a future."* WOW!! Rich, Cindy, Kirsten, and Kaitlyn sent me lovely flowers, and Linh Calhoun visited me for the last chemo and brought "chocolate fit for

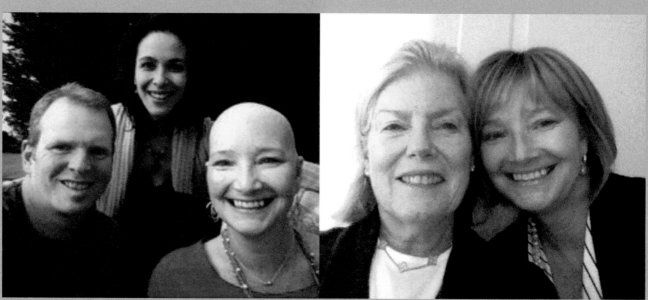

Me with Tom and Zully   *Me with Joan Litle*

a queen" and beautiful sunflowers and peonies. I am overwhelmed by everyone's love. As my good friend Maura says, "It's a love fest, and it feels great!" I agree. YOU ARE ALL THE BEST and I love you!

My focus for May is on rebuilding my strength, exercising, resting, and preparing for the big surgery on May 30th. I have chosen a bilateral mastectomy (double) and reconstruction. All will be fine, and I have plenty of loved ones coming to help me out!

Craig, my adorable HMN, is taking me to the Outer Banks to celebrate the end of chemo in mid-May. Craig has been fabulous, by my side the entire time, and I am SO grateful for having him in my life!! I love you, sweetie, and thanks for being there!!

I can't thank you enough for all your LOVE and SUPPORT. Your power circle of love has been amazing!! GET ON IT!!

Love to all,
Cindy Lou Who
Who has no more chemo :)

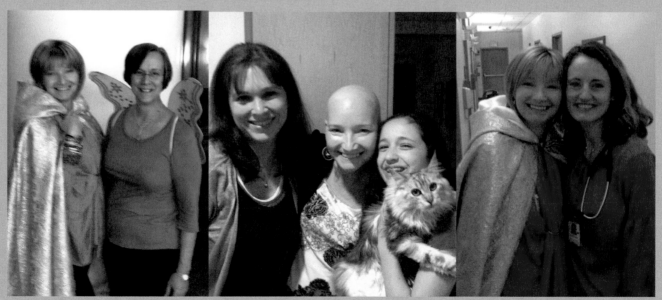

Me with Mary (AOE)   *Me with Stefanie and Elise Jandl*   *Me with nurse Anna Kate*

The outpouring of love was real and heartfelt. I even let others try on my "LONG AND LUXURIOUS" wig to experience what I feel like.

Chapter 12

CELEBRATING LOVE AND LIFE

Life goes on, and I got a month off from chemo! Woot! Woot! We CELEBRATED! We traveled to Maine to be with George and Fran for their annual Derby Day party. It was such a treat to see so many friends from Maine and L.L.Bean. The outpouring of love was real and heartfelt. I even let others try on my "long and luxurious" wig to experience what I feel like. George loved it the most! I rested as much as I could because my energy was low, but as I said before, April taught me to give in and let go. That's a freeing feeling.

Craig took me to the Outer Banks of North Carolina to celebrate the last weekend with my girls, my breasts. It was such a memorable weekend in so many ways. Perfect in every way! We drove the jeep on the beach. We packed a picnic lunch and found a private spot for cheese, crackers, and rosé. We explored Kitty Hawk, where the Wright Brothers first powered a flight in 1903. We ate lots of seafood and found fabulous restaurants for lunch and dinner. We had a very romantic weekend at the Sanderling Hotel.

DAY FIFTEEN POST-CHEMO

Written May 12, 2012 10:51 a.m. by Cindy Marshall

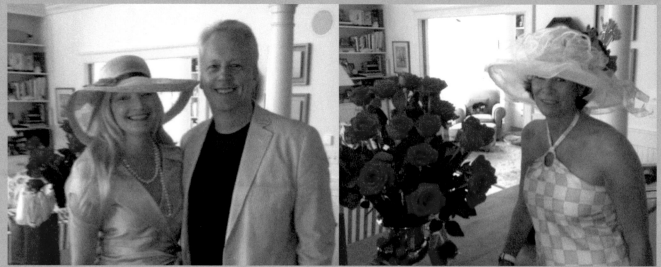

Me with Craig and Fran, Derby Day 2012

The doctors said it would take two weeks to get the chemo out of my system, so today is the start of healthy new beginnings!! I had strength last weekend while visiting friends in Maine and celebrating no more chemo, but this week I was more tired than usual. I am now expecting an upward climb to recovery as I build my strength and get ready for the big surgery on May 30th.

Since I last wrote, a lot has happened. First, I visited with Kali Bennert in Cumberland, ME. It was a treat to have quality time together. Kali is a close girlfriend whom I met when living in Maine during the late nineties. We did a lot of sailing together. Kali invited Kristen Moroney, Dorothy Holt, and Kristen Graffam King over for dinner on May 3rd and we had a great girls' evening! It was so great to reconnect with my girlfriends in Maine; it was as if no time had passed and we picked up where we left off. That's true friendship!! I even got to see Dorothy's husband Dan and their three kids for a brief hug and hello. The ladies even gave me a lovely pink, white, and blue scarf that I adore. Thanks so much, ladies. I love you all!!

Then I met up with Kim Noyes on Friday at Vicky's home for a spectacular lobster roll lunch! We had a great time, and it was super to spend time with Vicky in her beautiful home. Vicky is a great friend that I have known for seventeen years, and we have spent a lot of time together sailing, skiing, celebrating holidays, and entertaining. I am honored to have Vicky visit as one of my nurses after my surgery in June! Craig arrived in time for dinner, at which Fran outdid herself by serving a fabulous lobster mac 'n' cheese and mussels followed by Vicky's homemade key lime pie!! What a treat!!

Saturday was Fran's annual Derby Day party. It was a perfect day and evening. The party was fabulous— there were so many friends to visit with and delicious food and drink! Fran was dressed in a great jockey print from Vineyard Vines and a homemade hat topped with roses, a horse, a trophy, and winning money!

I received several gifts over the past week. First, Janice Izzi, my good friend from Vermont, sent me a Buddha necklace she had made for me from Santa Barbara—it's meant to heal and keep me strong. I love it!! Second, JD and Heidi, my brother and sister-in-law, sent me a care package with a healing candle, Pukka peaceful sleep tea (works great), and some socks! Third, Mel and Jerry Stoltz, Heidi's parents, and good friends, sent me a great book titled Laughter and Latte: Joyful Inspiration for Women, and cocktail napkins with a quote: "I'll have a cafe mocha vodka Valium latte to go, please!" Finally, Kim Noyes gave me a wonderful bracelet that she got at Abacus, a store in Freeport, that was handmade with love.

I also wanted to share some sad news. I spoke with my dad's sister on Monday, my Aunt Nancy, who will soon be joining other loved ones in heaven. I am so very sad, as she has always been a mentor of mine and someone I admire immensely. She is very young, in her mid-seventies. My cousins Christie and Julie are spending as much time as they can on Nantucket to be with her and Clark during her last days here. I am so grateful I was able to visit with both Nancy and Clark in March. I love you dearly, Aunt Nancy, and I send you strength, peace, and happiness!!

Onward and upward . . . I am focused on building strength as I prepare for the next stage of this journey, my surgery on May 30th. GET ON IT!

I love you all and thanks for your continued support!
Cindy

CELEBRATING AT OBX

Written May 18, 2012 6:55 p.m. by Cindy Marshall

Craig and I are having a fabulous time in the Outer Banks (OBX)! This is our post-chemo celebration trip, which began yesterday. We are staying at a fabulous place in Duck called the Sanderling Resort. We started our day off sampling Duck doughnuts, which are custom made to order, then walking the new boardwalk along the coast. After that, we went four-wheeling down the beach to Corolla, hunting for the wild horses and the perfect spot for an afternoon picnic. We found them both and had a ball driving down the beach in Craig's jeep. It was a bit breezy, but we managed to pick a sheltered spot in the dunes on a fabulous deck for shrimp, cheese, bread, and rosé! It was just perfect!!

I just came back from being pampered with a massage and pedicure at the Sanderling spa. Just what I needed to help clear out the last of the chemo. I am feeling stronger every day, close to normal—yeah!! No hair growth yet, but when it starts, I will be sure to share the mystery with you.

Thanks for your continued support!!

Much love,
Cindy

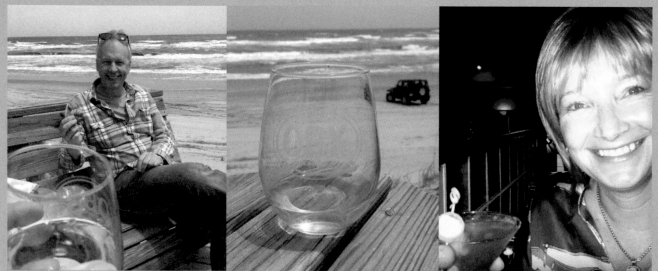

OBX picnic, beach cruising, and cocktails to celebrate

FEELING NORMAL AGAIN!!!

Written May 27, 2012 9:21 a.m. by Cindy Marshall

Yiippee!! I feel great: energy is coming back, and I am almost 100%. Craig even said he noticed changes in my energy level and other small things. I am so relieved to be feeling normal again. It's so hard to explain the chemo fatigue, but it's no fun. Last night Craig and I went to the UNC vs. NC State ACC baseball game in Greensboro and had a blast.

For all that don't know, I go on Wednesday, May 30th, for my bilateral mastectomy, and Fran is the first "angel on earth nurse" who will be taking care of me. Then Vicky, Barb, Heidi, and JD. Mary, AOE, will also be around to help with driving, airport runs, and whatever else is needed. And of course, Craig will be helping support everyone when he can. I am so grateful to my fabulous friends and family for taking the time to come help me out.

I will be in the hospital for two to three days, then home resting with my angel nurses. Fran and Craig will be keeping everyone posted on CaringBridge with the status of how I'm doing, so please check in when you can.

I love you all and thanks for your continued support!! I am close to reaching the bottom of the black hole and it's been a wild but good journey so far!! GET ON IT!!

Cindy Lou Who

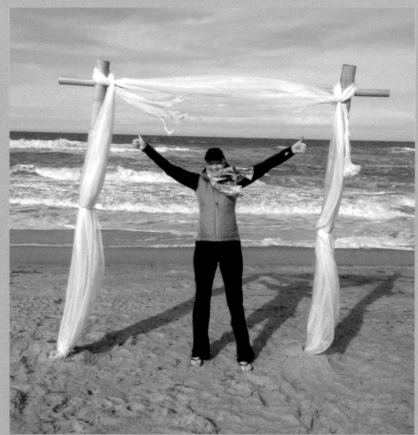

Me celebrating life at OBX

I can't begin to describe what it feels like to even think about amputating your breasts.

Chapter 13

TIME TO SAY GOODBYE

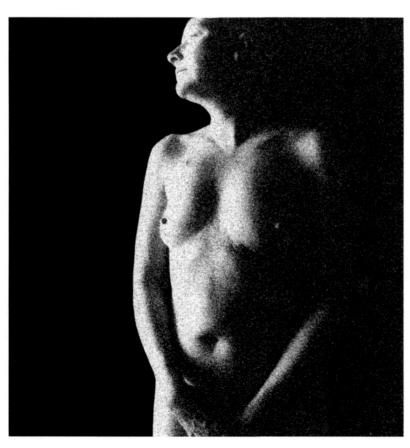

I can't begin to describe what it feels like to even think about amputating your breasts. Yes, that is what happened to me on May 30, 2012. I was so scared, but I didn't let others know this. I continued to be strong and treat this like it was a business project. Why? I guess that is how I was wired. But deep down inside, I was so sad and so scared. Our weekend away at the Outer Banks was good closure for me and helped prepare me for the big day. Craig and I talked a lot about losing my girls. We both cried and mourned the loss to come. We had many romantic moments together. We enjoyed delicious meals, romantic walks on the beach, and passionate moments in our hotel room.

A memorable moment was when Craig captured an incredible photo of my bald head and naked body in the 5 p.m. sunlight. The early evening glow was shining on me, and my face held the expression of sadness, yet strength to carry on. I realize now (nine years later) that I was stronger than I remember when I look at this image. I was also proud of my girls, and this was my way to honor them. This photo has since been turned into a painting by our good friend Wendy, which I gifted to Craig on his birthday in 2021. It is so special because it reminds me of what it was like to have natural breasts and nipples.

CANCER FREE TOMORROW!!

Written May 29, 2012 3:26 p.m. by Cindy Marshall

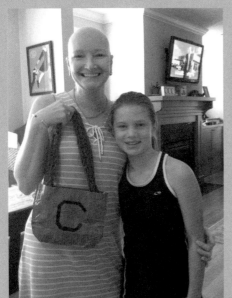
Me with Audrey Calhoun

To My Fabulous Circle of Power and Love,

You are all amazing and have helped keep me strong and positive through this journey of "kicking cancer's butt"! Tomorrow I will be CANCER FREE . . . I will be thinking of skiing Black Hole with all of you and screaming from the top of my lungs that I made it to the bottom! I know I still have some tough days ahead, but I am in a good place mentally right now. I am going to let the doctors do what they do best, trust in the good Lord, and let my fabulous nurses take care of me.

Craig and Fran are Team Cindy tomorrow. We check into the hospital at 8:30 a.m. and I head into surgery at 10:30 a.m. It will be a good five to six hours before they are done and I wake up. I am in good hands with Fran and Craig, HMN. I expect to be in the hospital for two to three nights, so most likely not home until Saturday, June 2nd. Craig's birthday is Sunday, and we are thinking of celebrating Saturday night with his favorite local BBQ, so I hope to be home for that! I also wanted to say thanks to a few folks for the latest round of gifts that arrived . . . I continue to be overwhelmed by the love coming my way. You are all amazing!

I am ready for the next step of this journey. I have had my tears along the way, but now I'm ready.

GET ON IT—onward to being CANCER FREE!

Love to all!!

Whoville

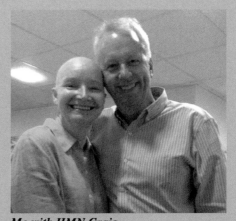
Me with HMN Craig

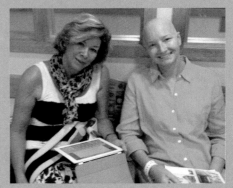
Me with Fran

SURGERY DAY

Written May 30, 2012 4:10 p.m. by Fran Philip

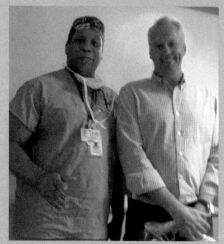

Dr. Amos and Craig

Craig, Cindy, and I arrived at UNC a little before 8:30, the scheduled check-in time. We spent the next few hours with Cindy as she got prepped for surgery and met with all the doctors and nurses one more time. At about 11 a.m., they wheeled her away. The first part of the surgery was to take an hour and a half to two hours, so Craig and I then headed to Merritt's so I could try the world-famous BLTs I'd heard so much about in some of Cindy's previous journal postings. The BLTs were indeed delicious. We then went home to make a few phone calls, walk Poppy, and get Cindy's things to bring to her room.

We were back at the hospital waiting room by 12:30, where a smiling Dr. Amos came out to see us after twenty minutes or so and informed us everything had gone very well. In fact, he called it "textbook" and "worthy of a training video!" Then it was time for the plastic surgeon, Dr. Halvorson, and his team to take over. In just a little over an hour, he came out to see us in the waiting room to tell us it went so well that it was "almost boring." Well, we like textbook and boring!

After about another hour and a half or so, Cindy arrived on her gurney outside the waiting room, and we joined the group taking her up to her room. She was awake and talking to us, wanting to know if we had had BLTs for lunch! She has a very nice private room in the east wing of Memorial Hospital. It is the corner room and so has beautiful light. She seems to be doing as well as expected and is just very, very tired right now.

POST-SURGERY DAY ONE

Written May 31, 2012 4:26 p.m. by Fran Philip

First of all, Cindy is so very grateful for all your guest book entries. She has enjoyed reading them over and over, so keep 'em coming! She really appreciates all the love and support.

She had an OK night last night. Did not get a lot of sleep, but that is really hard to do in the hospital! Dr. Amos checked in on her this morning and says she is doing great and all of the symptoms she is experiencing are very normal post-surgery, post-anesthesia issues. That doesn't make her any more comfortable, however.

Later on, a shower and fresh linens made her feel lots better. She has also been able to get up and sit in the easy chair in her room, as well as take a few short walks around the sixth floor. This afternoon, a very nice physical therapist stopped by to give Cindy an exercise routine to do at home for the next month or so. Luckily, many of the exercises are the same ones I have to do for my broken shoulder rehab, so Cindy and I will be able to do them together!

Mary Sullivan, aka AOE, stopped by for a few hours this afternoon. We are expecting another visit from Dr. Amos later today.

By the way, not only does Cindy have the best room in the joint, the food here is pretty darn good. She has about a twelve-page menu she can order from between 7 a.m. and midnight. There is Chinese food, sushi, BBQ, seafood, pasta, pizza, paninis, you name it! Nothing but the best for our girl. Tune in for tomorrow for our next set of adventures!

Fran

GOING HOME TODAY

Written June 1, 2012 2:37 p.m. by Fran Philip

Cindy had a great night's sleep last night and is resting very comfortably today in the hospital. She is really feeling 1000% better and looks great too. This morning we had another visit from the PT gal, who gave Cindy the award for the room with the most beautiful flowers. So thank you to Mary Lou Kelley, Leann and Paul Griesinger, Vicky Devlin, George Philip, and Debbie and Bob Dunkin for making that happen! Then we had a visit from Mary Norton, Cindy's next-door neighbor in Southern Village who works at UNC. And Mary Sullivan, AOE, stopped by for a couple of hours on her way to the airport to pick up Vicky, which gave me a chance to make a conference call.

But the best visit by far was this afternoon from one of Dr. Amos's residents, who says Cindy can go home today!!!!! So, we are now waiting for all the paperwork to be done and starting to pack up! I know the paperwork thing can take a while, but I am hoping to have our girl safe and sound at home by dinner time!

So thanks again for all your love and support. It really makes a difference!

Fran

No one told me what to expect or what the new normal would be like.

Chapter 14

ACCEPTING THE NEW NORMAL

What I didn't share in my journal was what a bitch I was when I woke up from surgery. No one told me what to expect or what the new normal would be like. I remember waking up from my surgery and all I wanted to do was see my breasts and see my scars. I demanded that the nurse show me, but she suggested I wait for the doctor, as there was no rush. I wanted nothing to do with that. I got so angry and belligerent. Craig and Fran were trying to calm me down. I was on so many drugs that I was irritable.

The nurse finally peeled back my hospital johnny to show me the damage. I was shocked because there were no bandages. I was so confused, because all I saw was a thin line with brown glue on both breasts and drains on each side. The nurse informed me that the plastic surgeon, Dr. Halvorson, used glue to seal me up. That was the first I heard of this, but I figured he knew what he was doing. I finally relaxed and waited for the doctors to come by to chat with me. UNC is a teaching hospital, so each time they visited, there were new students with them. I liked the idea of teaching, but I was also uncomfortable with the sensitivity of my surgery. Luckily, I loved my doctors so much that their presence relaxed me. Now it was time to think about living life without breasts and trying to figure out what the new normal was all about.

I'M HOME!!!

Written June 2, 2012 11:16 a.m. by Cindy Marshall

I can't tell you how wonderful it feels to be home!!! Fran did a great job capturing the hospital moments and of course has been the best nurse since I came home. I slept for a few hours when we first got home, then I woke up to the smell of bacon . . . yum, yum! Fran cooked a fabulous meal of pasta carbonara for dinner with a side of broccoli and a lovely salad! It was just perfect and made me feel even better. I even had a little ice cream. I slept soundly in my own bed—the pain meds and Advil helped. I was able to make it to the bathroom on my own a few times during the night. Fran said she checked in on me several times and I was out. I woke up to tea and a yummy smoothie by my side, thanks to nurse Frannie! I am resting in bed now after doing my PT exercises. All is as good as can be.

I can't thank Fran enough for being here!! Such a good feeling to be looked after by one of your best friends. Thank you, Fran!!! I love you!

My best friend and HMN Craig is on his way here to take care of me this afternoon. Then we plan to celebrate his birthday tonight with his favorite BBQ. His birthday is tomorrow, but the BBQ place is closed on Sundays. Vicky and Mary will arrive later today to join us in the celebration. I am feeling very blessed and loved.

Thank you all for your prayers, support, notes, flowers, and love!!!

Love,
Cindy Lou

DAY THREE HOME AND HAPPY!

Written June 4, 2012 12:10 p.m. by Cindy Marshall

Hi All,
Thanks for the continued notes of encouragement and love. I am doing well today, resting on the bed. I slept in and woke up to my new AOEN (angel on earth nurse), Vicky, handing me a smoothie and my morning tea! Vicky has taken over for Fran, who left early this morning. We are praying Fran has an uneventful trip home in the Nor'easter weather. I feel sooooo blessed to have such love around me!! Fran was amazing, and Vicky has stepped in without missing a beat. She even stripped my sheets today and remade my bed—wow, what

a treat—and now she is planning to make a fabulous homemade mac 'n' cheese for dinner!! Yum, yum comfort food!!

Yesterday was not a great day for me emotionally and physically, but I managed to stay strong to be with Craig while we celebrated his birthday! Such fun to watch the Diamond Jubilee activities in London—they sure know how to celebrate in style. Craig had a great birthday celebration on Saturday, and we continued on Sunday with leftover pulled pork sandwiches for lunch and a yummy crab cake, veggie, and salad dinner cooked by Fran!! No complaints here.

My emotional pain yesterday was due the news of losing my Aunt Nancy, who passed on to the heavens Saturday night. My heart was heavy and sad for her loss and the family she leaves behind. Nancy was an incredible woman who touched everyone with love and friendship. She was a role model and mentor to me, and I will always cherish the time we spent together, as well as everything she taught me. I know Nancy is resting peacefully in heaven.

I am so grateful for all of you!! Thanks for your continued love and support!
Cindy, aka Whoville

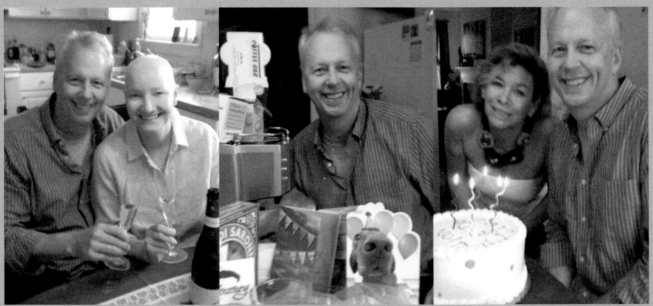

Celebrating Craig's birthday with Fran!

THE HOLY GRAIL!!

Written June 4, 2012 4:57 p.m. by Cindy Marshall

Yes, second post of the day . . . this one couldn't wait. I just received a call from Dr. Amos, my breast surgeon, to tell me the results of my pathology report, and I am completely cancer FREE!!! The margins are all clear—no cancer in residual tissue. Yippee!! This is what the doctors call "a complete pathological response" or as Dr. Amos says, "the holy grail of cancer treatment"! I am so relieved and so happy to know that we got it all and there is no more present.

The second bit of good news is that I get my drains out tomorrow at 1 p.m. YAHOO!! They are a bit painful and a big annoyance, so I am excited to have them out!

GET ON IT! Big canary wings have taken charge from above!
Love,
Cindy

A DAY OF THANKS!

Written June 5, 2012 5:46 p.m. by Cindy Marshall

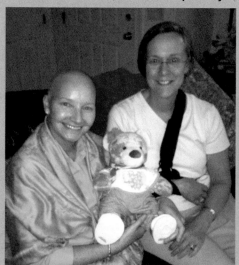

I am thankful to be free of cancer (YAHOO) and to be free of my drains!! I went to the plastics department today to see Nurse Sue Hayden, who is just a sweetheart, to have my four drains (aka turkey basters) removed!! Yippee! This is such good news on several fronts. First, I feel close to normal without carrying around drains filled with bodily fluid; second, it means my breasts are healing nicely with no infections; and third, I will be able to sleep better without rolling on top of drains. I am so relieved. One more step closer to being 100% healed (or should I say heeled for the Tar Heels). Sue also told me my scars are healing well and I look great.

Me with Mary (AOE) and Nunee Bear

Secondly, I am so thankful for AOE nurse Vicky Devlin, who took over for Fran on Monday. She has been a Godsend and is taking excellent care of me!! I wake up to fresh smoothies (thanks Fran for teaching Vicky how I like them), hot tea, and warm love. Then lunch and dinners prepared for me—last night we had her famous four-cheese mac 'n' cheese, and it was out of this world! So of course, we had leftovers today for lunch. Mac 'n' cheese is my favorite comfort food. Tonight, we are having a shrimp, coconut, ginger, and rice dish—yum!! Craig is on his way, and Mary Sullivan (AOE) is already here. What fun to have loved ones cooking for me. Vicky also does a great job making sure I do my PT and get the rest I need. Thank you, Vicky; you are a fabulous AOEN, and I love you!

I continue to feel blessed and loved by all. Thank you all so much!!
I love you!!
Cindy Lou Who

CHANGING OF THE GUARD (AKA AOEN)
Written June 10, 2012 1:36 p.m. by Cindy Marshall

Here I sit relaxing on a lovely Sunday afternoon waiting for my next AOE nurse to arrive—Barb Cozier, one of my fabulous sisters-in-law, who is married to my older brother Dave. She is arriving from Cleveland today, and Craig has collected her at the airport. I am looking forward to spending some quality time with Barb and grateful that she could be here!

This morning, Vicky and Sarah left to head home. Vicky was here for a whole week and was such a tremendous help!! She made sure I was fed well, resting, doing my PT, clean, and loved! I was spoiled by her, but it was just what I needed to help heal. I can't thank you enough, Vicky, for being here—you really helped me heal and I love you!!

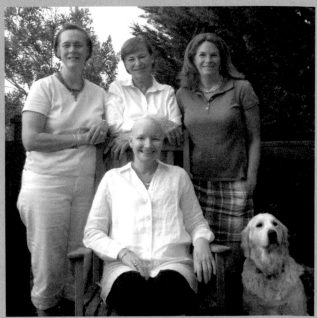

Me with Mary, Vicky, Sarah, and Poppy

Sarah, Fran's sister, came to visit on Friday. Sarah is like a sister to me, just like Fran, and they call me their adopted sister. Sarah is a beautiful woman, and it was so fun to catch up with her. She brought me a wonderful gift, handmade by a friend of her boyfriend, Chris. It's a wooden jewelry box that looks like a flower shed with a window. It is hand-painted in pink wash for breast cancer. It has a fall color theme, a pink ribbon on the outside, fall leaves, a black cat (for Jaguar, my kitty), pink velvet lining, a hidden compartment inside, and a canary to symbolize Stu Dog, who is an angel in the heavens watching over all of us. There were only four jewelry boxes made—one for each season—Vicky has Winter, Fran has Spring, and Sarah has Summer. I feel honored to have Fall! Sarah also decided to fix my front porch and plant a few flowers for me to enjoy. Thank you so much, Sarah. I love you!!

Mary Sullivan, my AOE, was also here almost every night for dinner while Vicky was here, since they are best friends. Mary brought me some new sunflowers mid-week to replace the ones in my guest room. She also cooked Thursday night dinner! In addition, she brought over "Nunee" who is her Build-a-Bear buddy that has been with her through thick and thin. Nunee came to show off her pink summer outfit and share some love with me. Thank you, Mary, for your continued love and support!! I love you, AOE!

The Pink Ladies of Vermont—Annette, Carol, Andrea, Lynn, Ellen, and Terry—gave me a "home massage." I was blown away! A beautiful young woman named Natalie arrived on Saturday with her massage table. She had a great spirit and was full of the perfect massage energy. The massage really relaxed me.

Daria, Eamonn, Saorise, and Clark sent me a goody bag of chocolate from Ireland and just ate two! Mary Ellen and Mindy sent me a Tempur-Pedic pillow!

Barb just arrived and she looks great. I am so happy to have her here. She brought me some Penzeys Spices from Cleveland. This is one store I have not visited, but apparently there is one in Raleigh. English Prime Rib Rub, Italian Dressing Base, Fresh Herbs, and Cinnamon. Can't wait to use these!

I continue to feel the love from everyone and it's wonderful. Thank you!!! I love the cards and the posts—keep them coming! Onward and Upward!

Love to all,
Cindy

FOUR WEEKS CANCER FREE!!

Written June 25, 2012 5:03 p.m. by Cindy Marshall

Hi All,

It's been a while since I last posted, mainly because I have been resting and didn't have the energy. It is now almost four weeks since my surgery, and every day I get better. Some days I do too much, which sets me back, but I am learning. I really want to be normal again, but as Dr. Amos told me last week at my three-week checkup, "Cindy, you had major chest surgery three weeks ago and you are doing great, but you need to give your body a chance to heal. It will take six weeks to feel better and be able to have more momentum. It will also take several months before you are fully healed. When I see you in six months, you will be a changed woman, and all will be great! Just be patient!" So here I go again . . . learning the patience lesson.

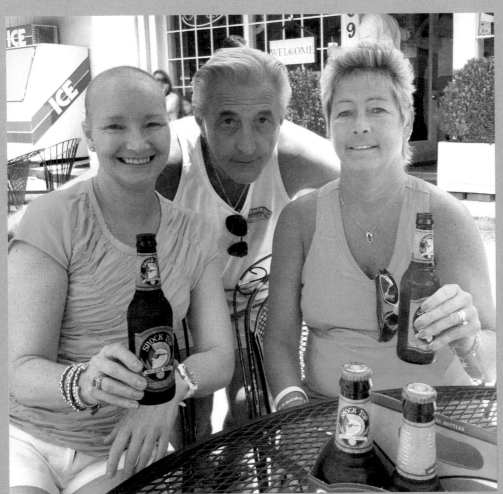

Me with Ivan Helman and Bonnie Kerlin enjoying BLTs at Merritt's

Last time I wrote, Vicky was leaving, and Barb was arriving here from June 10th to 15th and was a fabulous AOE nurse. She helped me a lot with cleaning, cooking, wash, shopping, driving, and resting. We had a

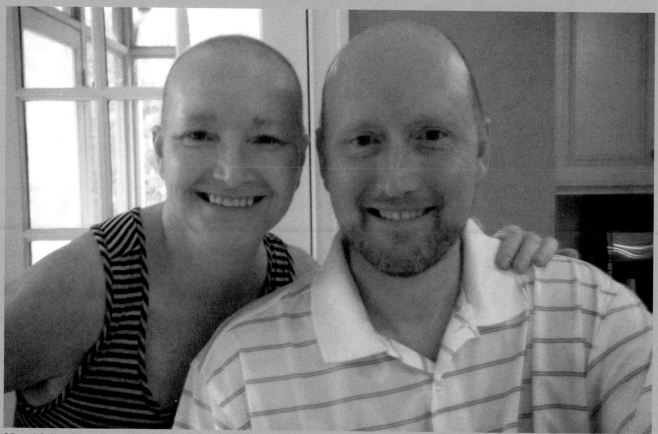

Me with brother JD

great time together bonding and sharing stories. Barb was just diagnosed with breast cancer a month ago, so it was helpful for her to hear what I've learned. The good news is that Barb caught it early and will be having a lumpectomy in early July. The bad news is that she has to deal with this cancer battle! But Barb is tough and has a very positive attitude right now. She is already a survivor and is coping well. I love you, Barbara, and I'm here for you. I am sending you love, strength, mojo, and prayers through this circle of power—the awesome friends and family we have on CaringBridge! GO KICK CANCER in the BUTT!

JD, my younger brother and twenty-five-year cancer survivor, came to visit on June 20th and left today. We had such a wonderful visit together!! I am so grateful to have had this time with him. He brought me some fabulous peppermint foot scrub and a natural body scrub brush as a healing gift from both JD and Heidi.

During his visit, we went to Craig's house in Greensboro and had a wonderful BBQ on Friday night. Craig and JD tried to play golf but got rained out. Then JD and I drove to Asheville to see our folks for Saturday and Sunday. We had a great visit. I rested a lot and JD helped them with clearing out books and fixing a bookshelf. It was so great to spend the time with them. We got home last night and then made four-cheese mac 'n' cheese for dinner!

JD has been terrific! He drove everywhere for me, got groceries, cooked, washed sheets, changed beds, emptied kitty litter and trash, and helped me rest. I love you tons, JD, and I am so thankful you were able to visit. Congrats on twenty-five years cancer free!!

Today I had a very special surprise: Bonnie Kerlin Helman and her husband, Ivan, arrived from Lake Havasu, AZ!! Bonnie is my best friend from elementary through high school. We grew up together in Potomac, MD, and did everything together!! We were glued at the hip and caused all sorts of trouble for our parents. My family was close with the Kerlins, especially since we lived a few streets away, so it's been fun to walk down memory lane together. Bonnie and I haven't seen each other for over twenty years!

Joan and Tim Litle sent me six pints of Graeter's Ice Cream in the mail! They arrived via FedEx in a dry ice box and were rock solid. Six flavors—vanilla, strawberry, mint chocolate chip, butter pecan, black raspberry chip, and mocha chocolate chip. Thank you!

Pam Higgins, my good friend that works at National Geographic, sent me a wonderful candle for the Hindu festival of lights—From Darkness into Light. She included a write-up about the light, and this is my favorite part "From darkness until light—the light that empowers us to commit ourselves to good deeds, that which brings us closer to divinity." Thank you so much, Pam!

I received beautiful flowers from Craig's mother, Jeanne, and her best friend, Yvonne, who live in Salisbury, England. The flowers arrived the week after surgery and were absolutely beautiful—purple, yellow, and white—all my favorite colors. Thank you so much, Jeanne and Yvonne!

I received a new set of flowers this week from Margot Murphy Moore, a very good industry friend and former NEMOA president. These flowers arrived in a yellow vase and had a yellow-and-white theme. Thank you so much, M3!!

Daria sent me some arnica gel, arnica pills, and another French cream that is meant to heal scars. It's very special because it came from Ireland, and I don't think it can be found here. I have been using it daily and so far, it's working wonders! Thanks Daria—I needed this!!

I've also received more cards. It means so much! I love you all and thanks for your continued support!

GET ON IT!
Cindy Lou Who

GRATEFUL

Written June 28, 2012 11:37 p.m. by Cindy Marshall

I'm grateful for today! I'm grateful for all of you, my family and friends! I'm grateful for having Craig in my life. I'm grateful to reconnect with so many people I care about! I'm grateful to have visited with Mary Ellen Hart today, one of my very good friends from Vermont who now lives in Lexington, KY, and came to visit me in Chapel Hill. I'm grateful to have chatted with Mindy, Mary Ellen's wife, on the phone tonight. I'm grateful my hair is growing back—all over my body! I'm grateful to be me and to be alive!

Grateful . . . what a great word. I recently lost a very special woman in my life, my Aunt Nancy, who passed away on June 3rd. I spoke with Uncle Clark yesterday to check in because I wasn't able to make it to her celebration of life on June 16th at the Nantucket Congregational Church, but my brothers Dave and Rich attended. They said it was incredible and the perfect tribute to Nancy.

When I was speaking with Clark, he offered to share the memorial sermon with

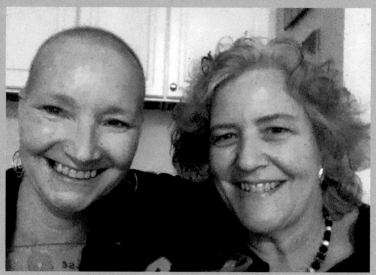

Me with Mary Ellen Hart

me, which I read today. The reverend described Nancy as "determined, generous, and grateful." Nancy was all of these and more . . . she was a mentor to me who taught me about grace, love, and how to deal with life's difficult challenges. I truly believe her passion and determination for life has helped me get through the past six months. Thank you, Aunt Nancy, I LOVE YOU!!

After reading the sermon, I continued to think about the word grateful all day, so I decided to share my grateful thoughts of today with you. I can think of a ton of things I'm grateful for this week . . . Craig, JD, Bonnie, Ivan, Mary Ellen, BLTs, interviews, family, rest, Jaguar, being cancer free, etc.

I want to sign off with a few quotes from Nancy's celebration of life . . .

DETERMINED, GENEROUS, GRATEFUL . . .
that is how Nancy will live on in the hearts of those who loved and knew her best.

"I have fought the good fight, I have finished the race, I have kept the faith." = DETERMINATION

"Whoever wishes to be great among you must be servant of all." = GENEROUS

"Rejoice always, give thanks in all circumstances." = GRATEFUL

LOVE to all!!
I'm grateful for you!!
XOXO

I remember how tight my skin felt on my chest.

Chapter 15

BUILD-A-BOOB

As I began my second month post-mastectomy, I started to realize that I was building my boobs, and I was fascinated with modern technology! I was grateful for having a malleable human body that could react, heal, and rebuild as time passed. I called the summer of 2012 my "build-a-boob summer." First, I learned how to give in, rest, and relax. I said no to doing things, going out, or simply doing household chores, which was hard for me. I let Craig pamper me and take care of me. This was a treat.

Second, I focused on building my boobs with my first appointment three weeks after my surgery on June 18th. I went in to see the plastic surgeon so they could fill my boobs with fluid to stretch the skin. During my surgery, I had expanders placed in my chest wall underneath my muscle. My skin was too tight, and my breasts were too small to have "same stage reconstruction," where they remove the bad breast tissue and insert implants. Each expander has a port attached to fill with fluid. I remember the doctor telling me how many cc's of fluid they were inserting, but that didn't mean anything to me. I was a 34B before I lost my girls, and I decided I wanted to have slightly larger C breasts. Based on this, the doctors knew how much fluid to give me. We waited two to three weeks after each treatment for the skin to expand to the enhancement, like how a woman's body expands with pregnancy. I had my second expansion on July 5th and my third on July 26th. We decided to have one more expansion mid-August for C-sized breasts. This meant I would wait one month for implant surgery, where they take out the expanders and replace them with implants.

I remember how tight my skin felt on my chest. It hurt for about a week as the skin expanded. When I reached the final size, I was a little freaked out, because my new fake boobs were hard and didn't feel good. It was like having half a grapefruit taped to my chest for each breast—the same hardness. I didn't feel sexy, that's for sure. They were ugly-looking with a big scar across each breast and no nipple. Dr. Halvorson, my plastic surgeon, kept reminding me that these were temporary. Thank God that was true. The implants feel closer to normal but never 100% real.

Meanwhile, I was interviewing with brands and trying to determine the next phase of my business life. I had to do something, as I really missed work. It was great to be back in person with all my NEMOA friends and leading the NEMOA organization as the president and chair of the board. I had started interviewing with National Geographic for a marketing consulting role in April and May. Of course, I put everything off to recuperate from my surgery during the month of June.

SIX WEEKS CANCER FREE!! YAHOO!

Written July 12, 2012 11:23 p.m. by Cindy Marshall

The doctors told me I would feel normal at six weeks, and thank goodness I do!! The six-week point is when stitches have fully dissolved and the body has healed for the most part, meaning full range of motion. Two days ago, I was able to fully reach above my head and put dishes away—that was huge for me. I now have a much better appreciation for the purpose of our pec muscles; they are critical for many everyday activities. I am off all meds—yippee—and only taking Advil at night if needed. Such a relief!! I can't do a downward dog or get on my bike, but soon I will.

Since I wrote last, I had a wonderful visit with my good friend Mary Ellen Hart, who lives in Lexington, KY, working for Tempur-Pedic. It was such a treat to see her!! We visited on the evening of June 28th when she was in town for work. She surprised me with a martini glass that is hand-painted with pink ribbons and the words friend, mother, daughter, sister, and promise. Thank you, ME, for visiting—it was so nice to see you—and thank you ME and Mindy for the wonderful martini glass. Now we need to share some cosmos in person!

Craig and I spent the first weekend of July in New York City visiting with family and friends (sorry to miss you Sid, Curtis, Bill, and Talbot). On Friday night, we had a spectacular dinner at Bice with Craig's brother Mark and family—Mary, Suzie, and Chris. It was such a treat for me to meet Suzie and Chris in person—I've heard so much about them!! We had a nice lunch on Saturday with my good friend Jan Cantler and her husband, Will, at Fig & Olive. That was a special treat! Then we met up with Jon and Vicky Baxter-Wright, for a tour of MoMA and a nice dinner at Rockefeller Center. Jon and Craig were good friends in high school and haven't seen each other for over thirty years, primarily because Jon and Vicky live in Australia. On Sunday, we had brunch with one of Craig's good friends, Kate Marber, and her friend Chris, who was visiting from London. Kate has been a huge supporter of mine, and it was such a treat to finally meet her in person! It was a magnificent visit to the city and a delight to connect with Craig's family and friends!! Needless to say, I was very tired come Sunday night . . .

We spent July 4th, and the weekend following, relaxing by Craig's pool, swimming, reading, and BBQing . . . a perfect way to help recover! This week, I've been busy with work interviews and exploring options for my next career move. I feel fortunate to have options and to reconnect with many industry friends.

I continue to be amazed by the love and support I've received during this journey. Your continuous positive attitude has kept me focused and upbeat during this fight, and I thank you for all you've done for me!! I recently took all the cards and special notes I've received from YOU and glued them onto hot-pink paper and put them into a three-inch pink binder!! It's quite impressive and something I will cherish forever.

I will leave you with a short story from today. I live in a small Chapel Hill community called Southern Village, where you can walk to the local shops for all your needs. Over the past year, I've gotten to know the shop owners of Strays general store, Babara and Bob. They have followed my progress each week and encouraged me to carry on—they even helped me select my favorite wigs. Today, Barbara told me that I have been such an inspiration to her that she wanted me to have a special gift that was given to her. It's a handmade breast cancer bracelet with pink ribbon beads, pink ribbon, and love and hope charms. The woman who made it wore the bracelet during a breast cancer walk for her friends and family. Barbara passed it on to me with love and wants me to continue to pass it on to other women when I feel the need. It was such a surprise and such a special treat, it brought tears to my eyes. I don't even know her that well, but I guess I've made a difference in her life, just like she has in mine. I plan to wear the bracelet, along with all the other ones I've received, this October in the Charlotte Avon cancer walk.

Thank you family and friends for your continued support!!

All my love,
Cindy Lou from Whoville
GET ON IT

OFF TO LONDON—YAHOO!

Written July 29, 2012 9:17 p.m. by Cindy Marshall

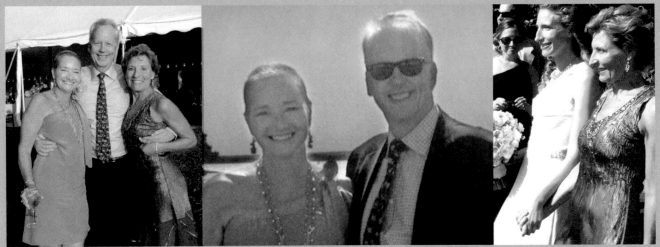

Me with Andrea and Craig at Jessica and Mark's wedding

Hi Beautiful Family and Friends!

WOW! Just seven months ago, it was December 2011, and I was diagnosed with breast cancer (shock and fear) and went through massive tests (pain and unknown future), but doctors said I could travel to Ireland for Christmas (visiting Daria, Eamonn, Sairose, and Clark) and London for New Year's (with my HMN Craig). Last time I left for the UK, I didn't know what the future would bring me. I didn't know my treatment plan (chemo and/or radiation) or my surgery plans. It's hard to believe that I went through four months of chemo and a double mastectomy. WOW!!

Tomorrow I travel with Craig to London to visit with his family and good friends for a week. I am so excited and happy to be cancer FREE this time! We will be staying with Chris and Deb Reynolds, Craig's best friends, for the first part of the week, and then off to Salisbury for the balance to visit with his Mum, Jeanne Waller. Jeanne turned eighty in June, and her entire family (less one) will be in England to celebrate—how fun! Craig and I were fortunate enough to get tickets to the Olympic tennis match on Wednesday. We have center court seats at Wimbledon!! We are both so excited!! We are hoping to visit the Olympic Village sometime toward the end of the week. Craig will be doing the "roof walk" of the 02 Arena with his daughter Chloe on Thursday, which should be a special treat for them! I will report back after our week in London.

In the meantime, I feel the urge to update you on the past two weeks. Now I am eight weeks cancer free! HA HA! Loving every minute of it and grateful for life. We had a quiet July 4th in Greensboro, as I was still recovering. I have to say swimming in Craig's pool has been so helpful. We went to Bristol, RI, for Jessica and Mark Mazzenga's wedding this past Sunday, July 22nd. Jessica is the daughter of Andrea Diehl and Rob Steuer, good friends from Bennington, VT. I adore Jess and was thrilled to be included.

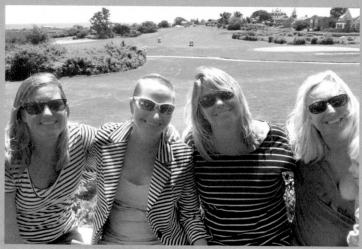
Me with Stephanie, Katie, and Karen

Before the wedding, we stopped in Westport, MA, to see Cosmo (Karen Desantis Flather) and her lovely family, Buck, Kayden, Ashton, and Cole. It was such a treat, as I hadn't seen them for maybe five years, way too long. Cole is three years old, and I had not met him yet. It was fabulous to see them all, and then Cosmo surprised me by inviting good friends and ski buddies Stephanie and Katie to lunch. So I had to include a photo of the babes!

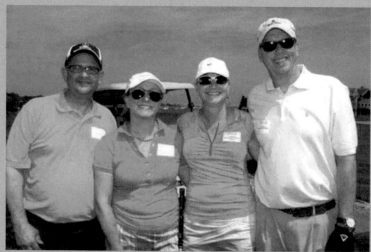
Me with Todd, Margot, and Craig

On Monday, July 23rd, my brother Richard's birthday, we drove to Rye, NH, to NEMOA's twelfth annual golf event. I was able to play golf—didn't do well, but had fun! We had eighty people turn out for our event and it was a magical time—perfect weather, perfect venue, great food, and excellent company! The NEMOA board decided to raise money for cancer research, so the theme was "Wear pink!" We had pink golf balls donated by Wiland Direct (thank you, Phil, Brent, and Dan) and pink towels donated by Brightcloud Marketing (thank you, Karen).

Speaking of Brightcloud, Karen Jordan, the owner and a longtime industry friend, gave me a lovely silver bracelet that I will cherish forever! It was truly an honor to see everyone wearing pink, and we raised over $2,500 for breast cancer research.

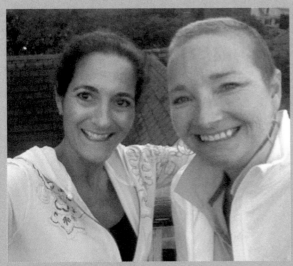
Me with Maura Maloney

On Tuesday, I visited with Maura Maloney, a good friend of mine whom I have known since college. Maura is a four-year breast cancer survivor and doing great! It was wonderful to share stories and reconnect!! Maura treated me to a fabulous dinner on the seaport and then a nice evening on her condo roof deck!

On Wednesday, I spent the day with good friend Leann Griesinger in Boston. We had lunch upstairs at Sam's overlooking the Boston skyline and harbor. Leann gave me a book called *Slow Love* written by Dominique Browning, the former editor of *House and Garden*. I am loving the book—it's just what I need to continue to inspire me to write my own story. Dominique writes about losing her job, putting on pajamas, and finding happiness. I can relate! I remember meeting Dominique, along with publisher Brenda Saget, when I worked at eZiba, because we advertised with them. I just looked up my business card file and there is her card!!

YOU ARE MY CIRCLE of POWER and YOU helped me KICK CANCER's butt! Thank you everyone!!

GET ON IT!!
Love,
Whoville

BRILLIANT DAY AT WIMBLEDON!!

Written August 2, 2012 5:59 a.m. by Cindy Marshall

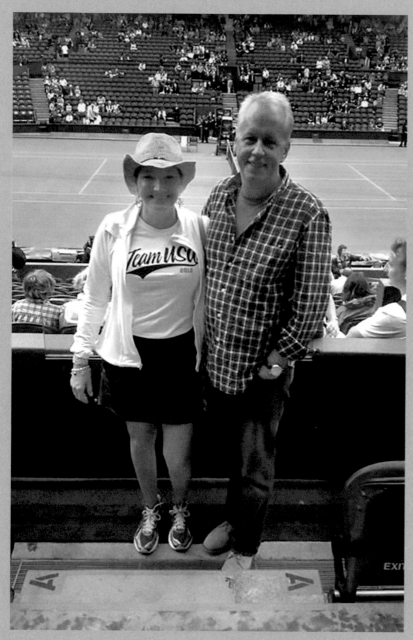

Reporting in from England . . . Yesterday was a perfect day!! Chris, Craig's best friend, drove us into Wimbledon from their home in Godalming (south of the city) and dropped us off at the gates—nice service!! Chris works in Wimbledon Village, so it was very convenient. Our tickets were in Centre. We watched Serena Williams from the US beat Vera Zvonareva from Russia. Serena is so strong and so talented; her serves measured 150 km/h in speed! Then we watched Djokovic beat Hewitt, which was an intense game and a very close match. The men's serves were 190–200 km/h in speed! Wild!! We had Pimm's and a banger for our first snack and then we decided to sit down for lunch after touring the other courts. Our afternoon was spent watching Britain's Andy Murray beat Marcos Baghdatis of Cyprus in a very thrilling and close match (4–6, 6–1, 6–4). This was the men's semi-quarter finals. The crowd went nuts!! It was spectacular, but William and Kate never showed up. At least I saw the royal box! Craig even saw Federer's wife while shopping—way cool.

We walked to Wimbledon Village at the end of the day to meet Chris and then ended the evening with a fabulous BBQ cooked by Deb and Chris! We even had a lovely Opus One wine, which Chris was saving for a special occasion! It was a perfect day all around!

Have a great week and GO TEAM USA!!
Love,
Cindy

MY HAIR IS GROWING!

Written August 24, 2012 1:41 p.m.
by Cindy Marshall

Just a quick update. I am in Vermont now, visiting with friends, and spent the earlier part of the week with Williamstown buddies. I will post photos of this week's adventures later but today I wanted to share my new hairstyle—it's growing and is now blond! My hairdresser cut a little around the ears and the neck, but the top is as is . . .

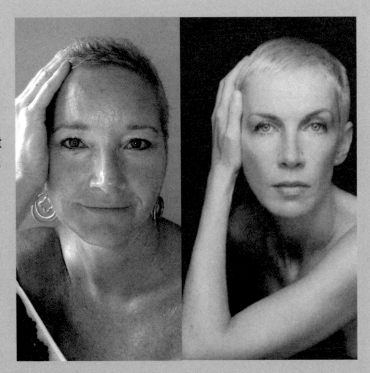

Almost close to Annie Lennox—check it out!
Love to all!
Cindy

PS: having a ball spending time with all my buddies in Williamstown and Vermont!!! I do miss it here!

WONDERFUL WILLIAMSTOWN

Written September 3, 2012 7:57 p.m. by Cindy Marshall

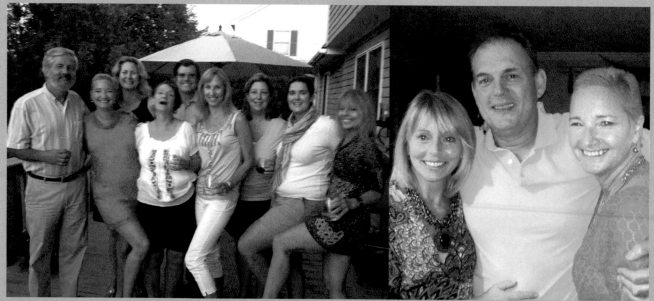

Me with Williamstown friends at Cindy and Paul Poulin's

Hi All,

I have a lot to update you on with all my travels the last few weeks, so you will see several journal updates.

I spent a week in Williamstown, MA, and southern Vermont doing my "walk of honor," as Craig calls it, visiting with all my pals. My primary reason for the trip was to spend quality time with my fabulous friends who gave me so much love and support during my fight. It had been fourteen months since I last visited Williamstown or Vermont, so it was time.

On Tuesday, August 21st, Cindy and I went to Caretaker Farm to pick fresh flowers, veggies, and berries for our dinner. It was truly a treat and made me wonder why I was never a member of Caretaker Farm when I lived in Williamstown. It was a special experience and one I will cherish. That evening, Cindy and Paul Poulin hosted a wonderful and delicious "farm to table" dinner party for me at their house in Williamstown. It was such a treat to see everyone; it filled my heart with joy. Thank you to Alix and Brian Cabral, Suzanne Farley, Jane Patton, Emily Eakin, Mary Edgerton, Tom Greenwood (Annie too), and Cindy and Paul for a brilliant evening!!

On Thursday, I had a nice visit with Jane and Emily and their beautiful twin girls, Olivia and Addison, at their house. I can't get over how adorable and grown up they are! Then Jane treated me to a lovely lunch at the Taconic Golf Course—what a great spot! That afternoon I took off to Shaftsbury, VT.

Thank you to all my Williamstown friends. I love you tons!!!
Cancer Free Cindy Lou Who
GET ON IT!

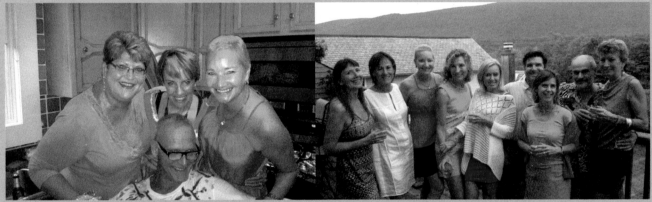

Me with Kathy, Janice, and Sid   *Me with Vermont friends, too many to name*

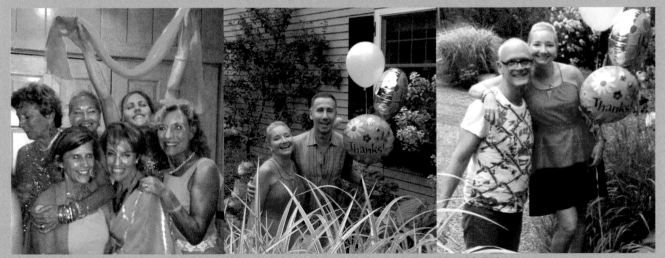

Vermont Pink Ladies   *Me with Curtis*   *Me with Sid*

VIBRANT VERMONT

Written September 5, 2012 10:33 p.m. by Cindy Marshall

On Thursday night, August 22nd, Andrea Diehl and Rob Steuer hosted a dinner party at their house in Shaftsbury, VT, so I could see some of the pink ladies (Ellen, Terry, and Lynn). It was another memory-filled evening with lots of laughs and delicious food! Thank you, Andrea and Rob, for spoiling me with good cheer, fab food, yummy wine, and great company. I know Rob enjoyed being surrounded by five lovely ladies. HA!

On Friday, Andrea, Terry, Zues, and I hiked the trails at Park McCullough House in North Bennington. Early in the afternoon, I took off to Manchester and visited with Sheila Sullivan and her adorable son Tanner. Then a quick stop at the Vermont Country Store offices to say hello to Geof Brown, Chris Vickers, and Annette. I ended up at Curtis and Sid's lovely Manchester home for the next several nights. We visited and got caught up, then Janice arrived to bring me a gift and visit—such a special treat. On Friday night, Sid and Curtis took me to Al Ducci's new restaurant for dinner—delicious Italian!!

Saturday the 25th, I spent a relaxing day catching up and getting ready for our big BBQ party that night. I went to yoga with Curtis, did a little shopping with my personal assistants, ate lunch out, took naps, and prepped for dinner. Sid and Curtis hosted a party for many of my Manchester friends. It was an amazing evening, and I am still smiling from all the fun. It was a group effort; everyone brought a dish (lots of desserts), The best part was that everyone wore inspirational pink. I loved it!! It was a special time for me to give back and say thank you to my Vermont friends that supported me with love and strength during my fight. I even wore my chemo cape at one point to share with the Vermont Pink Ladies who made it! It was truly a magical evening and thank you, Sid and Curtis, for hosting. You ROCK! A BIG THANK YOU to everyone who made the party—Janice, Lyman, Kathy (fifteen-plus-year breast cancer survivor), Vince, Tamara, Michael, Malc, Carol, Terry, Annette, Andrea, Ellen, Lynn, Tony, Stephen, Ronda, Adam, George, Jeff, Tom, Greg, and Judith. Sorry to miss others that were not around or couldn't come.

On Sunday, Janice called and said, "Let's go to the Dorset Farmer's Market," so Sid, Curtis, and I joined Janice at the market, and we had a blast. It was a real Vermont country experience and I just loved it! Then we went to Carol's house to visit for her birthday and eat some of the leftover cake from the night before! Tony, Lynn, Terry, and Andrea were already there visiting, so it was an extra special treat to see them again.

Malcolm and Carol live on a beautiful piece of property in Dorset and are preparing for a bonfire party on September 21st (my final reconstruction surgery date), so we decided it would be an ideal spot for photos. WHAT FUN!! More quality time was had by all! But we didn't stop there . . . the ladies decided to visit Annette to see all the hard work she has done in her gardens. We totally surprised her, but she was a trooper and stopped working to show us her orchards, bees, and many gardens—truly spectacular and an inspiration to us all!

Are you tired yet?? Still more visiting . . .

Sunday afternoon, I went over to Terry's A-frame house in Rupert and relaxed on the deck (yes, I needed it). She has an amazing view, and it was a lovely day, the perfect way to end the day. Terry cooked a healthy meal for me and Annette, who joined us after her hard work in the garden. We had a very nice evening, but I collapsed at eleven . . .

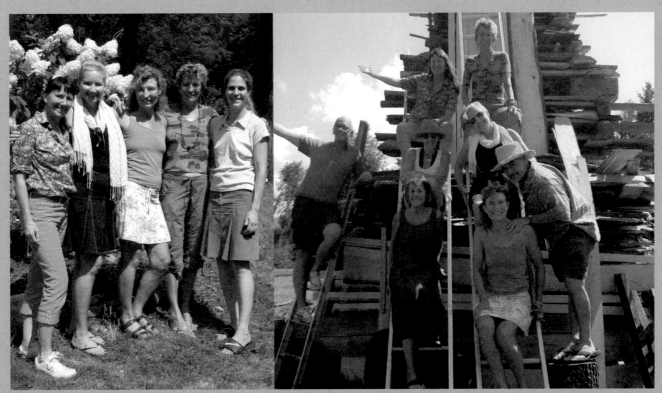

Me with Vermont friends at Malc and Carol's

Monday started out early, off to breakfast at Sherry's Cafe in Manchester with some of my former colleagues from VCS—Judy, Julie, Sheila, Janet, David, Donnel, and Annette. Great quality time and good for me to see them all doing so well!! I sure do miss my friends and colleagues from VCS! Donnel was kind enough to walk me through the halls of VCS after our breakfast, so I could visit and see what had changed. I caught up with many people and it made me happy to see them all! I then visited with Laura Hain, my former neighbor, at her office in Manchester (Parks and Recreation Center). It was great to see her and hug her! Then I took a trip south to Shaftsbury and had a quick visit with Bob and Helen Hain, my friends and former neighbors. We had a great visit with lots of big hugs. It was odd to be back on Holy Smoke Road next to my old house, but there was a sense of closure for me to see the Shaftsbury house and know that life has moved on. There were

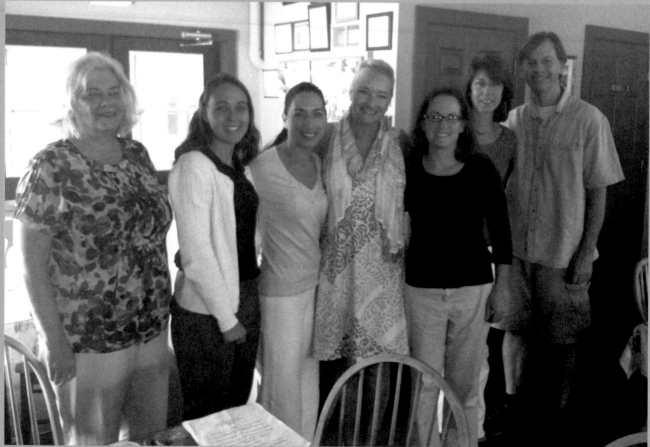

Me with former team from Vermont Country Store—Judy, Janet, Julie, Sheila, Donnel, and David

many great memories at that house, and memories never die—they stay with us, which makes us who we are. I ended up at Andrea's house to do some work before heading to the airport. Yes, I was tired. I sure slept well that night when I got home.

THANK YOU everyone for making my trip so special!! I love you all!
GET ON IT
Cindy

PS: Please send love, prayer, mojo, strength, and support to my sister-in-law Barbara as she goes through the breast cancer fight. She started chemo today, the first of four treatments. Then she will have radiation. I am sending her the circle of love to help her heal!! I love you Babs and you will be FINE!

I wanted to do something to help fight the battle and be part of a movement to stop breast cancer.

Chapter 16

SHINE ON!

SHINE Strategy was born the summer of 2012 and was officially incorporated in August, when I signed on for a three-month project with the National Geographic e-commerce team. I started the process of talking to Nat Geo in April. This three-month project turned into a three-and-a-half-year contract and became the foundation for my strategic consulting business, sometimes referred to as Chief Marketing Officers for hire. The three-month project was to develop a three-year marketing road map that drives revenue and profit growth based on historical trends and new initiatives. After I delivered the road map, Nat Geo asked me to stay on to help execute the plan. I was beyond delighted!! This road map became a proprietary tool I developed called the SHINE Road Map, which I continue to use today, ten years later. We look at media spend and performance results for a two-year period to project three years of revenue and profits.

In April of 2012, I remember flying to DC during my chemo to meet with the senior executives at Nat Geo to discuss how I could help them. Of course, I wore one of my seven wigs, my favorite short and sassy one, the one I wore to meet the postmaster general. I recall the flight attendant on the plane telling me that she loved my haircut, the color, and the shine! That was a sign . . . I was beginning to shine. This simple message helped me begin to feel somewhat normal. I let her think it was my hair the entire flight. When it was time to disembark, I felt dishonest, so I finally broke the news to her that it was a wig, and I was going through chemo for breast cancer. She was blown away and hugged me! I felt so empowered and loved.

At the time of launching SHINE, I wasn't sure I was made out to be a consultant, because I loved leading and teaching teams, plus my extroverted personality needed daily interaction and challenges. It took me about six months to realize that I was great at being a consultant and I had a lot of knowledge to offer in terms of performance marketing and growth plans for multichannel retail brands. Being a consultant allowed me to have more "thinking time" because I wasn't dealing with office politics. This insight was eye-opening and recharged my drive to succeed. My business quickly began to grow. I signed my second client—Southern Season, a small retailer in Chapel Hill—in September, and my third client—Boden USA—in October, with whom I worked with for eight years. Yes, at that time I was going through the recovery process of my "build-a-boob" summer with expanders, my implant swap surgery in September, and trying to regain my strength from all the meds, anesthesia, and surgeries. Somehow, I succeeded, and I am proud to say SHINE Strategy, which Craig named, is still successful today, ten years later.

I decided to take a stand to "get on it" and fight for cancer in October 2012, Breast Cancer Awareness Month, especially having lived through eleven months of hell. I teamed up with Heather Keets Wright, a co-worker of Craig's who was diagnosed a month after me. Heather had been doing some content work for the American Cancer Society and suggested their Making Strides Against Breast Cancer walk in Charlotte on October 24, 2012. We GOT ON IT and team Heather and Cindy raised $8,877, thanks to all our amazing family and friends who supported us! We ended up being team number four out of 214 teams!

The other thing that is so powerful about this breast cancer walk was that Heather and I had never met in person until the night before the walk. During the prior ten months, we became close breast cancer buddies through phone and email. We talked constantly and shared our stories each step of the journey. Heather is a remarkable soul and a true gift on this earth!

MAKING STRIDES BC WALK—NEED YOUR SUPPORT

Written September 6, 2012 11:59 a.m. by Cindy Marshall

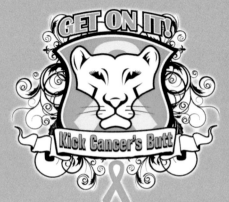

Hi All,

Another update—this time I need your support. On October 20th, Craig and I will be participating in an American Cancer Society event called Making Strides Against Breast Cancer in Charlotte, NC. We are joining forces with a good friend, Heather Keets Wright, another breast cancer survivor, to raise money to support other women. Please support us—join our team with a donation and/or come walk with us!

Our team is called Heather and Cindy, GET ON IT.

As many of you know, I decided to attack the breast cancer fight just like skiing the "Black Hole" run at Sunday River. WHY? Black Hole is the most difficult double diamond at Sunday River, ME—it's challenging, exhilarating, and scary, yet you eventually conquer it and reach the bottom of the trail, the end. I remember the first time I skied this trail; I was standing at the top with several ski buddies, and everyone was looking down the hill, scared. They kept waiting to go, so finally I said, "GET ON IT," and took off down Black Hole!! After that, Stu Dog Jones continued to call out to me "GET ON IT, Whoville." It has stuck with me for over fifteen years, so I decided this would be a good motto for attacking breast cancer. It worked—I am now 100% cancer free after four months of chemo and a double mastectomy!

I decided to dedicate this Making Strides walk in honor of Stu Jones. He passed away last Thanksgiving, and it was at his funeral that I decided to have my breast pain checked out (Stu was in angel mode). He taught me how to GET ON IT! Thank you, Stu Dog. I love you!

Please help Heather, another breast cancer survivor, and me raise money to support other women.

We are planning to have T-shirts made with this logo. More details to follow!

Much love,
Cindy

PS: Today I had my four-month check up with oncologist Dr. Lisa Carey and Dr. Anna Kate Owens. They said I was doing great, and they loved my short sassy hair; they called it CHIC! They also said I had "complete pathological response," which means my tumors were killed by the chemo!! They said this is the BEST place to be, and they celebrate this. YAHOO!! I knew my margins were clear but didn't realize the chemo killed all of the tumors!! GET ON IT!

LABOR DAY IN PORTLAND AND VANCOUVER

Written September 22, 2012 4:42 p.m. by Cindy Marshall

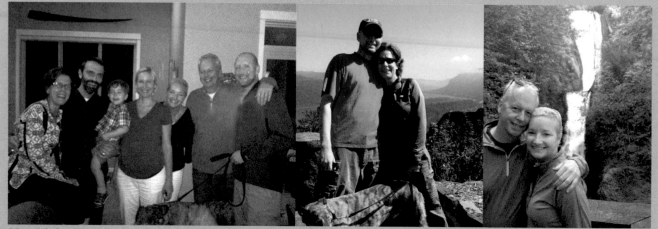

Me with family at JD and Heidi's home

Yes, I know, I'm a little late writing about Labor Day, but I've been busy! Craig and I went to Vancouver, WA, to visit JD and Heidi (my brother and sister-in-law) over Labor Day, and we had a blast!! It seems like so long ago . . .

JD and Heidi treated us like royalty with action-packed days, sightseeing, and amazing meals! Best of all was relaxing together in their beautiful new home in Vancouver—very comfortable!!

We did a lot and not in this particular order. We toured downtown Portland, visited the Japanese Garden and the Rose Garden, had a yummy brunch at the famous Screen Door Restaurant (owned by cousins Nicole and David Mouton), had a delicious lunch experience at Clyde Commons, had dinner and delightful wine at Higgins, hiked along the Columbia Gorge, had drinks at the Skamania Lodge, took a private tour of the Nike

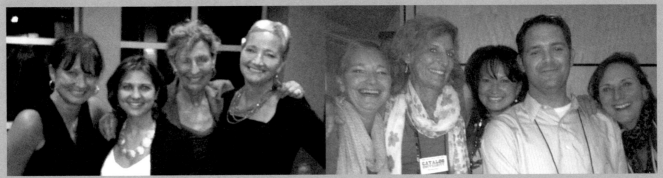

Me at NEMOA with Linh, Heather, Andrea, George, and Nancy

offices (thanks to Craig's good friend Barbara Frank, who works there), went shopping at the Nike Portland store, went shopping at Art in the Pearl, and ate amazing meals at JD and Heidi's, including a fabulous BBQ on Sunday night with David, Nicole, Henri, and Barbara. It was truly wonderful. JD and Heidi, THANK YOU for all you did to make our trip memorable and full of special moments. We love you!

I just got back from our fall directXchange conference by NEMOA in Mystic, CT (this is the organization I am president of). It was a lot of work but also a HUGE success!! I am grateful for the NEMOA staff members, Terri and Kris, and our board members, who made it run so smoothly. I am also grateful to have so many wonderful friends in the industry; it truly feels like family every time we get together! We also had a special guest from the American Cancer Society who was present during my opening remarks. We presented her with a check for $2,385, which was the money raised at our annual charity golf event! Very moving!

My daily reading for Thursday, September 20th, from *The Book of Awakening* by Mark Nepo, was about unconditional love. I want to leave you with this saying because this is how I felt during the NEMOA event.

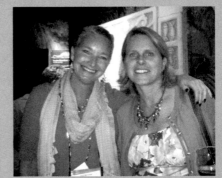

"Unconditional love is not so much about how we receive and endure each other as it is about the deep vow to never, under any condition, stop bringing the flawed truth of who we are to each other."

GET ON IT!!
Love to all,
Cindy

Me with Pam Higgins, Nat Geo

ONE MORE STEP TO BEING DONE!

Written September 25, 2012 10:59 p.m. by Cindy Marshall

Hi All,

Many of you have asked, so I decided to update my journal. Tomorrow I have outpatient surgery at UNC for my second-to-last reconstruction phase. This is when I get my "real breasts" that will be much more comfortable and softer. Dr. Halvorson, my plastic surgeon, will swap out my "breast expanders" that were used to stretch my skin for my permanent silicone implants. I can't wait; I am SO done with the skin expansion thing.

I am told it's a very easy procedure and not painful like the first surgery, because the muscle has already been cut and the nerves are less sensitive. Angel on earth, Mary, will be picking me up at 6:15 a.m. (ugh, better get to sleep) for a 6:30 a.m. hospital check-in. The good news is that I will be first in line and should be home midday. It's a two-hour procedure and then time to wake up. I am sure I will be groggy tomorrow afternoon but should be back to feeling normal by the end of the week. Craig is in Toronto at the headquarters of his client, Four Seasons, for business meetings. He is so bummed he can't be here, but with me in spirit! Originally my surgery was planned for Friday, September 21, but it got moved to tomorrow due to the doctor's schedule. GET ON IT already!

Tomorrow is also Barbara's second chemo treatment and halfway mark. She had a tough time with low white blood count during week two after her first chemo and was in the hospital at Cleveland Clinic for a week. YUK! She has shown incredible strength, and her spirit is bright and cheery despite the setback. I just ache for her and pray that tomorrow goes much smoother. This time, she will be taking Neulasta, the white blood cell booster shot, which helps a lot! It saved me. She also shaved her head today and she looks fabulous!!! GO BARB!! GET ON IT Sista!

So I ask all you—this powerful circle of strength, love, and mojo—to surround Barb and me tomorrow with your prayers as we both continue on this breast cancer journey.

Much love to all!
Cindy

PS: More to follow later this week about my new business, SHINE Strategy . . .

SUCCESSFUL DAY!

Written September 26, 2012 9:27 p.m. by Cindy Marshall

Hi All,

Just a quick update to let you know surgery was a success and I've been home resting since 2:00 today. Mary Sullivan, my AOE, has truly shown her wings today!! I couldn't have done this without her. She picked me up at 6:15 a.m. We got checked in and ready for surgery by 8:00, when Dr. Halvorson came to draw all over me (he called it his version of Mona Lisa). We had several very handsome doctors wait on me, including Dr. H. That made our morning! I got my pre-surgery "cocktail" at 8:15 and was wheeled away. I barely remember the operating room. Woke up around 12 or so but not sure . . . had a great nurse, Margot, prepare me to go home.

When we got home, Mary AOE had stocked my house with comfort food from Whole Foods!! God bless you, Mary!! She also picked up two beautiful bouquets of flowers—one from Vicky with beautiful antique hydrangeas and other lovely-smelling flowers, and sunflowers from Fran and George. Absolutely gorgeous. THANK you! Craig sent me two thoughtful cards, which arrived today! Then Mary tucked me into bed, and I was out cold. Mary went home to let Harry out and came back at 4:00 with my Vicodin meds, fed me, and tucked me in again. I slept from 5:00 to 8:30, which was great. Dr. H told Mary I needed rest to keep the sutures in place, so I am being like a cat and sleeping all day! Off to read and back to sleep for the night.

Thanks for your love and prayers!! They worked!!

Love,
Cindy

HAPPY SUNDAY!

Written October 14, 2012 4:21 p.m. by Cindy Marshall

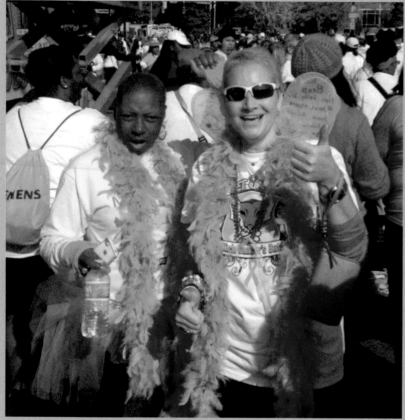
Me with Heather at finish line

Hi All,

Just a quick update to let you know I am doing well post-surgery. I was very sore for a good week and rested for the three to five days following surgery. I forgot what general anesthesia does to one's body . . . definitely knocks you out and makes you feel bloated. I saw my doctor on day ten post-surgery and he was very pleased with my new girls. He informed me that he wasn't 100% happy with them so he gave me extra anesthesia to do some more work to center them! Glad that Dr. Halvorson is a perfectionist! I am pleased with them, and they are healing well. Still a little sore, but Advil helps with that.

Heather and I have about twenty people walking with us; we are so excited! We even have some good friends flying in from LA to walk, Larry and Bruce!! We have a lot of pink stuff to wear (boas, hats, beads, face paint, etc.) along with our GET ON IT T-shirts. We plan to have a lot of fun—pictures to follow after the event!

Enjoy what's left of this beautiful Sunday!

Love,
Cindy

THE FINISH LINE!!

Written October 24, 2012 9:11 p.m. by Cindy Marshall

Hello Wonderful Circle of Power and Love!

We did it! We kicked cancer's butt and we crossed the finish line healthy!! This past weekend was our walk for Making Strides Against Breast Cancer in Charlotte, NC. Team Heather and Cindy raised $8,877 thanks to all of you!!! We were team number four out of 214 teams—holy cow! I would say that we GOT ON IT and it is because of all of you. Thank you for supporting us!

Our group was at least twenty-five people . . . not quite sure of the final count. I do know that the total walk had over five thousand people!! It was very impressive and very moving.

Heather is a four-week cancer survivor and for me it's four months!! We wore survivor bells on our shoes and signed the survivor banner. It was an incredibly emotional and memorable time for me. I have to say this was closure for me. I'm DONE with this cancer stuff!! Crossing the finish line was a great symbol to remind me of that. Now all I want to do is help others survive.

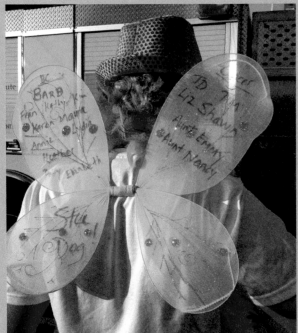

You will notice that I wore angel wings during the walk. On the left wing I wrote all the names of women I know who have survived breast cancer—Barb, Fran, Kim, Maura, Karen H, Karen B, Lydia, Kathy, Annie, Heather, Patty, and Elizabeth. On the right wing I wrote the names of other cancer survivors—JD, Liz, Shawn, and Tim. I also wrote down the names of my Aunt Emmy and Aunt Nancy, who recently passed. I forgot my cousin Michelle on the wings, but she was with me all the way. I also wore every bracelet and necklace that people gave me during my fight, so everyone was with me!

Our shirts said GET ON IT—Kick Cancer's Butt. Very cool to see everyone wearing GET ON IT shirts. Thanks to Heather's good friend, who designed the logo!

My wings—walking for others

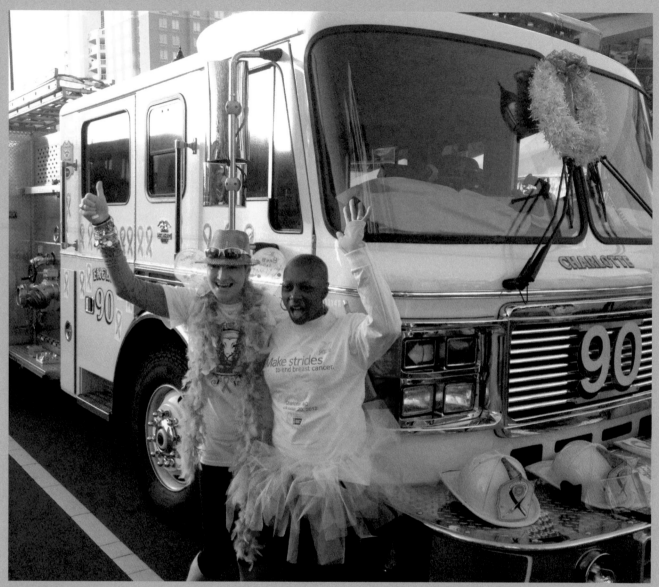

Me with Heather

Michelle Mohr, a friend of Craig's from US Airways, and Larry Williams, a good friend from work, walked with us. It was so great to have their support. A big thank you to both of you! After the walk, we had lunch with Larry before he went back to Greensboro.

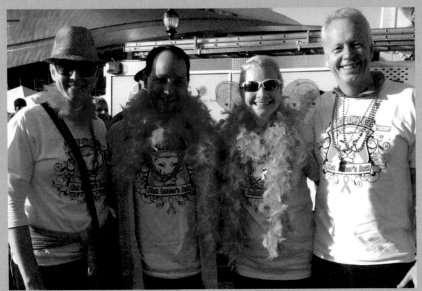
Me with Michelle, Larry, and Craig

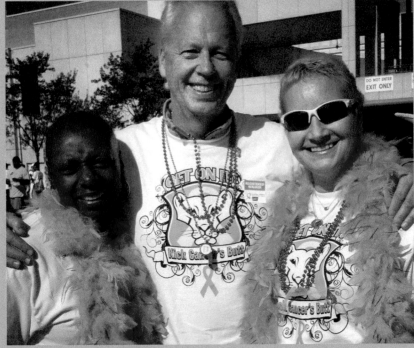
Me with Heather and Craig

Sunday morning we met Heather and Mark (Heather's fabulous husband), along with Dr. Amos (my amazing breast surgeon) and his wife and three girls for brunch at Mimosa in Charlotte. It was a real treat to see Dr. Amos outside of the hospital being a father and loving husband. After brunch we all walked to the football stadium to see the Dallas Cowboys play the Carolina Panthers. It was a glorious, sunny, blue-sky day! The game was great. Panthers almost won but Dallas scored in the fourth with three minutes left, and we lost . . .

But the weekend was a BIG WIN!! One that I will remember forever! Thank you all for helping me walk the finish line with pride and joy! We did it—we KICKED it in the butt!

Much love to all,
Cindy

Now I have new nipples . . .
but they are just for show to help
me feel more normal.

Chapter 17

ALL I WANT
FOR CHRISTMAS IS . . .

Yes, all I wanted for Christmas were my two front nips! This sounded like a song, but it was another surgery. UGH. This time I had two doctors who did the surgery, the lead surgeon and an intern who was going to UNC Chapel Hill. I didn't know when I went under that each one would take a breast (is this why we have two breasts?). The intern watched the surgeon do the first nipple and then he practiced on the other breast. They described the process to me as taking a three-inch sliver of skin and wrapping it around itself to form the nipple. There's an eighty-plus percent chance it will stick, but there was a chance the blood flow will get cut off and the nipple will turn black and fall off. Thankfully, my nipples stayed put.

When I went back for post-surgery checkup, I asked why they looked so different, and that was when they told me the intern did one and the surgeon the other! Now I had new nipples . . . but they are just for show to help me feel more normal. In three months, I went back and got areolas tattooed on. I had to do that twice to get the color I wanted, and that process was another story.

Craig took off to England for Christmas to be with his family, and I went to Freeport, ME, to spend the holidays with Fran and George. It was a very moving holiday for me because so much had happened in the past year. It was also very emotional because it was at Fran and George's home that I received several messages loud and clearly, "If you think there is a lump, go see your doctor." If I hadn't listened to that message, I would not be here today. These messages came from Shawn McKeena, Liz Cook, and Kim Noyes. Sadly, Shawn and Liz both lost their battles with cancer a few years later.

On December 23rd, Fran and George hosted a party in my honor for my birthday and to celebrate seven months cancer free. There were twenty-eight people who attended, including many friends I hadn't seen in a long time. I was overwhelmed with joy, love, and gratitude. There was even a Whoville toast written by Shawn for me that was meaningful and very funny!

I went to church on Christmas Eve and cried with joy surrounded by friends who loved me, sang Christmas carols, and rejoiced at being alive. Life was a gift! It was so remarkable to me to think about the past year and to be alive to celebrate it. This message has stayed with me every day. I believe nothing else matters but family, friends, and love!

DAY ONE OF A NEW HEALTHY YEAR!

Written December 9, 2012 11:48 a.m. by Cindy Marshall

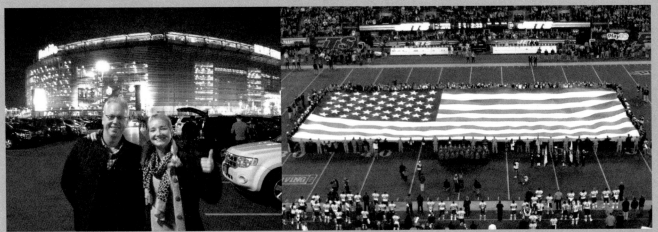

Photo on Thanksgiving Day at MetLife Stadium for the Patriots vs. Jets game with the CT Waller family

Hello Everyone and Happy December!

Yesterday was the anniversary of the day I was diagnosed. It's not something to celebrate, but as I reflect on the past year, I can't get over what has happened.

Diagnosis on December 8, 2011, medical appointments, Christmas in Ireland, New Year's in London, decisions on treatment, lymph node surgery, chemo port surgery, four months of chemo, lost my job, trip to the Outer Banks to celebrate end of chemo, double mastectomy on May 30th, recuperation, learning I was cancer free, a summer spent stretching my skin with breast expanders (not fun), a London visit for the Olympics (!!!), launching my own business in August, celebrating cancer free with MA and VT friends at the end of August, implant swap surgery on September 26th, recuperation, American Cancer Society breast cancer walk in Charlotte (thank you!), back to life as I once knew it (not really . . .) and finally on November 30th I celebrate six months of being cancer free! YAHOO I'm done and moving forward!

WOW. Even I am tired thinking of all that happened. It was a tough year, but thank God it's behind me. Today I start a new year and a new life of being healthy! I was on a five-month wait list to get into Get REAL and HEEL at UNC, which is an after-care breast cancer program, and I received a phone call on November 28th that I was in! The REAL stands for Recreation, Exercise, Active, Living. My breast surgeon (Dr. Amos) and my oncologist (Dr. Carey) both recommended me for the program, and I am so excited to get started. Get REAL and HEEL is not just an exercise program. It integrates individualized prescriptive exercise with recreational therapy to provide a program that strengthens your body and mind. It's supported by grants, so it's free for breast cancer patients. I had a cognitive assessment on Friday; next week I get my physical assessment; and in the new year I begin the program with other breast cancer survivors and will go three times a week. This will help me get my body back in shape! It will also help me connect with other women dealing with the same issues post breast cancer.

Many of you know that I started my own business called SHINE Strategy in August. Craig came up with the name SHINE, which I love. My icon is a sunflower, as it makes me happy. SHINE Strategy provides retail consulting to help brands increase sales and profits. I have been working with National Geographic (the online store and catalog) since August, and I'm really enjoying the team and the work. I started working with Southern Season, a local retailer that specializes in gourmet foods, wines, housewares, cookware, and unique gifts. I also started working with Boden, helping the marketing team in the US and M.LaHart and Company, a collegiate marketing brand. Plus, I've been busy with my NEMOA presidency role, planning our spring conference. No grass is growing under my feet.

I have a lot to look forward to in 2013, which will be my fiftieth year, but not until the end of the year. First, I get my "nipples" on Tuesday, which is the last medical procedure I have to deal with. It sounds funny to say out loud but it's the final touch, like putting frosting on a cake! In the new year, my plastic surgeon is moving to Boston to work at Brigham and Women's Hospital so I wanted him to finish his work of art, plus I wanted to feel physically normal for my forty-ninth birthday on December 27th! Bring it on!

Next weekend, I visit my folks in Asheville to have an early Christmas and attend my dad's SAR (Sons of the American Revolution) luncheon. I am looking forward to seeing them! On December 19th, I head off to Maine to be with Fran, George, Vicky, Kim, and many others for the Christmas holiday. Fran and George are throwing a party on Sunday, December 23rd, in my honor, which gives me the opportunity to celebrate life with all my Maine friends! So excited! We also hope to ski a few days at Sunday River. YIPPEE!

I will spend my birthday with Craig in Chapel Hill, and then we head to Hilton Head for a long and relaxing New Year's weekend.

I am most excited about being alive and living every day to the fullest—that is what it's all about! I give thanks to all of you for your support this past year; I couldn't have done it without you! You are my circle of love, power, mojo, prayer, and strength! I am very GRATEFUL for all of you!!!

Much love,
Cindy

HAPPY CHRISTMAS!!

Written December 25, 2012 3:31 p.m. by Cindy Marshall

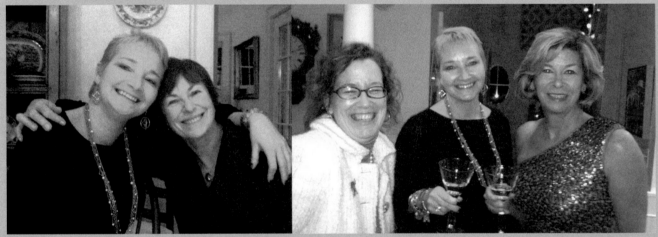

Me with Vicky, Kim, and Fran

Dear Loved Ones,

I wanted to send a quick note to say Happy Christmas to all of you!! Thanks for your continued support and love this past year! I am so grateful to be here and to have conquered this past year!

I am having a wonderful time in South Freeport, ME, at my good friends George and Fran Philip's home, which is a beautiful spot on Brigantine Cove in Casco Bay. This morning we woke to the magical sight of snow falling all around, a delightful gift from above! Vicky joined us for Christmas breakfast and several hours of gift opening. I feel like a part of the family—very special! We even had Jambo, Fig, Max, and Heidi (their furry kids) help open gifts.

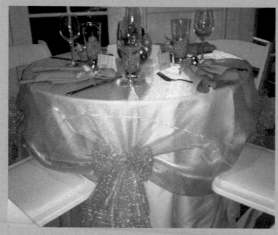

Last night, we went to two open houses followed by an incredibly delicious dinner at Tony and Denise McDonald's and finished the evening at the 10 p.m. Christmas Eve service at the South Freeport church. My favorite part is singing Christmas carols, especially "Silent Night" by candlelight, and celebrating the birth of Christ with everyone at church!! Very special!

On Sunday, December 23rd, Fran and George hosted a party in my honor for my birthday and to celebrate seven months cancer free! There were twenty-eight people that attended, many of them friends I hadn't seen in a long time. I was thrilled to see Liz Cook, who has been battling liver cancer for eighteen months. She is a real survivor and looked amazing!! I was completely overwhelmed by all Fran and George did to make this a memorable evening for me.

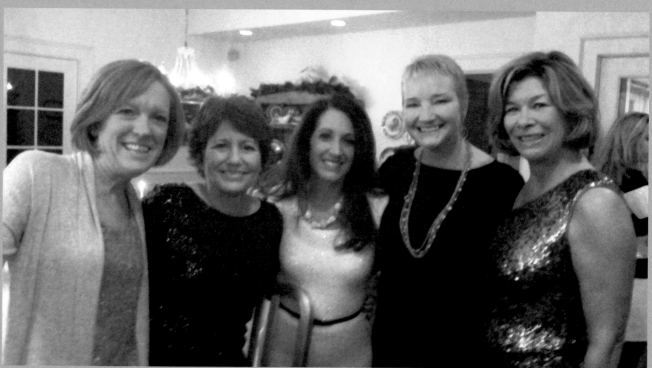

Me with Jill, Liz, Kristina, and Fran

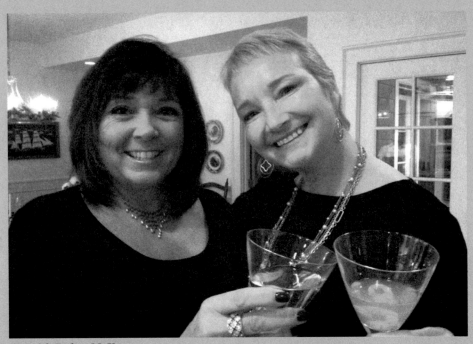

Me with Debra McKenna

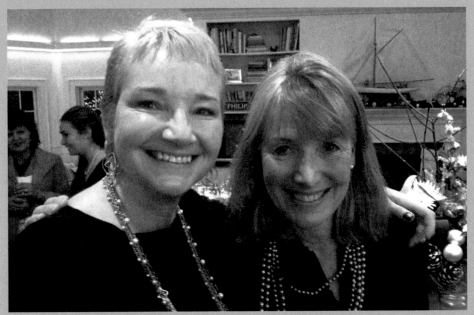

Me with Kathleen Bernard

There were many surprises, from Whoville Martinis with peppermint candies to Cindy Lou Who cookies and cake. The house was dressed to the max with a blue and silver theme—very elegant and extremely festive. The sit-down meal was catered by Evelyn and crew with delicious hors d'oeuvres and a spectacular beef bourguignon!! WOW. It was truly over the top, and I am so very grateful and thankful to have such amazing friends like Fran and George!! I love you guys and thank you for all you did for me!

There was one more surprise from the evening, which was a toast that Shawn McKenna did for me. It was so moving that I had to share it with you.

Shawn is a cancer survivor (just over a year!) and a huge supporter of mine. Thank you, Shawn. I am grateful for you!!

TITLE:

Cindy Lou Who . . . and the Grinch That TRIED to Steal HER Christmas

Note: Grinch is synonymous with cancer in the toast

TOAST:

We gather here to honor our friend, Cindy Lou Who

She has just gone through almost a year of much "to do."

When we were asked to think of some relevant words, perhaps even a toast, we felt we needed to reflect the grit of Cindy and also that of our hosts.

So it made sense for us to (short form) retell Cindy's story, one that would make most wince and revel at the fact that she put the smack down on the no-good SOB Grinch.

Every Who down in Whoville likes Christmas a lot, but the Grinch who lived just north of Whoville did not!

Fast forward . . .

And the Grinch grabbed the tree, and he started to shove, when he heard a small sound like the coo of a dove. He turned around fast, and he saw a "smoking hot who"; it was the shapely Cindy Lou Who, who looked like she was thirty-two!!

The Grinch has no sympathy—it is impartial and it does not care—and he unleashed his discontent on Cindy Lou Who, oh one so fair.

But he did not have any idea, not even a clue, at the focused resolved of one . . . "Cindy Lou Who."

The Grinch and life itself attacked this indomitable spirit and gave it its best, but Cindy would not succumb, would not bow, and continued to live and fight for life with her own special zest.

It went after her body and ohhhhhh what a fine body it was; it unleashed its savagery and turned her beautiful hair into "peach fuzz."

Cindy Lou Who fought back with a steely resolve; her body took some hits but her spirit did not dissolve.

So we gather here tonight to honor you, Cindy Lou Who. You are amidst friends who unreservedly love you.

You did not just endure, you did not just survive, but you lead by example, you have fought the good fight, and we thank God you are alive!!

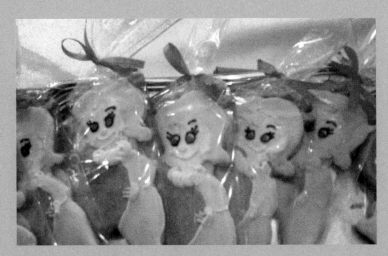

WOW. This is what life is about—family, friends, and love! Thank you, everyone! I am grateful for you all and feel blessed to be here! Happy Christmas to all!

Love,

Cindy Lou Who

I was tired of doctors, tired of commuting between Chapel Hill and Greensboro, tired of feeling like shit, tired of everything.

Chapter 18

GET REAL AND HEEL

The new year, 2013, arrived and life began to feel very hectic. Craig and I were both very busy with work and exhausted from the past twelve months. We wanted life to get back to normal. But what was the new normal? I was tired of doctors, tired of commuting between Chapel Hill and Greensboro, tired of feeling like shit, tired of everything. I was learning how to live my life with a new body, a new job, and low energy.

One of the best things about UNC Chapel Hill was their breast cancer resources. I never felt alone. I joined a group called "Get REAL and HEEL" (for the Tar Heels), which met two to three times a week for exercise and once a week for nutritional and emotional discussions. This was one of the best things that happened to me during my recovery. I met so many amazing women and realized I was part of this new tribe called breast cancer survivors (now called thrivers). We all understood what the others were going through. They paired groups of breast cancer patients together that were at similar stages, yet we all had different types of breast cancer.

I want to share a story with you that made me realize I was extremely lucky to have this amazing support group of family and friends. I learned that many women go through this alone and don't have anyone or a group of people to lean on. One of my survivor tribe friends told us that she never told her husband she had breast cancer because she was terrified that he would leave her. I didn't understand this—how could you not tell your partner and lover in life? She bought a wig that was exactly like her hair so that she could go through chemo without him knowing. She also kept it a secret from her job and coworkers. She took time off work for chemo treatments. I understand why people can be afraid of losing a spouse or a job (and many do), but this is your life, and only you can choose how to live it. Get rid of the fear. Let it go. Seek help to get you through. Share with your closest partner in life. If they can't understand, they are not meant to be your partner in life.

Before cancer, I was a Chief Marketing Officer for a $250 million dollar cycling business with over a hundred stores. I was an avid cyclist, and I rode with some amazing cyclists and former racers. I was very active. I skied, I hiked, and I did yoga all the time. I had no idea that it would take years to recover physically. I remember the nurses telling me it could be five to seven years, but of course I didn't believe them. I didn't want to hear this, so I blocked it out. I was being a selective listener! Now that I look back on my post-treatment recovery, it did take me at least five years to bounce back to feeling fit and energized again.

Get REAL and HEEL clearly helped me get over the fear of exercising again. By the end of January, I was starting to feel stronger, and I was in a routine that helped me stay motivated. This new normal was difficult to accept, but I kept powering through. I was looking forward to Valentine's Day, especially because Craig and I think of it as our first official date in 2010.

HAPPY VALENTINE'S DAY!

Written February 14, 2013 3:44 a.m. by Cindy Marshall

Happy Valentine's Day to My Fabulous Circle of Love!

Wow, what a difference year makes . . . I am so thankful to be eight and a half months cancer free and to have 2012 behind me!

I loved giving Valentine's Day cards during my childhood . . . remember those cute little packages we could buy with fun valentines?? Each page would have a collage of four to six images. I guess they would be considered "vintage" now. During elementary school, I loved giving cards to everyone in my class—what fun that was!! And of course as we got older, wanting a certain boy in class to give us a special valentine . . . or giving "secret" valentine cards . . . oh the simple days of youth!

In the spirit of giving, I'm sharing something I learned from my Get REAL and HEEL program. They taught us two breathing techniques to help deal with "stresses" in our daily lives. The first one is called "Quick Coherence Technique" and the second one is "Attitude Breathing Technique." Both are designed to help you focus on "happy thoughts."

QUICK COHERENCE TECHNIQUE

Step 1) Heart Focus

Shut your eyes, relax, and focus your attention in the area around your heart.

Step 2) Heart Breathing

Imagine your breathing coming in and out of your heart area. Visualize your heart in your chest beating up and down. Breathe slowly into a count of five seconds and breathe out to a count of five seconds. Continue this breathing pattern until your breathing feels comfortable and rhythmic.

Step 3) Heart Feeling

Continue with the heart breath and focus on a positive feeling, thought, or image that brings you a sense of love or gratitude. Continue focusing on this thought while also continuing the heart breath and the heart feeling. Visualize this love feeling around your heart . . . and now your stresses will be gone!

Spread your love and sunshine to all! Happy Valentine's Day!!

I Love You,

Cindy Lou Who

I was sad, angry, and confused.
I didn't understand why this was
happening to me.

Chapter 19

CAN'T DEAL

February and March were tough months for me. I was hit with a flew blows that would break my heart and my bones. During this time, Craig and I were struggling as a couple. Valentine's Day would mark our three-year anniversary of our first date, but for half of the three years, I was sick and dealing with treatments and surgeries. Craig was a total saint and never gave up. He was by my side the entire time. He was my savior and my hot male nurse! He supported me through everything, even when I was no fun to be around.

I wanted to move in with Craig. I wanted to have my life partner with me, and I wanted to get married, even though I had failed at it twice before. This time was different because I had found the right partner for the rest of my life. Well, none of this was coming true. In fact, the opposite was happening—we were slowly separating. My heart was broken. I was sad, angry, and confused. I didn't understand why this was happening to me.

I needed to prove to myself that I was strong and that I was loved. I would say to myself, "If Craig doesn't want me, then it's time to move on and live my life on my own." Of course, that was the opposite of what I wanted. Given this mindset, I decided to book a trip to Vermont to see my posse of girlfriends. Andrea and Rob were celebrating their 120th birthday on March 2nd, when they would turn sixty within days of each other. I couldn't miss this celebration, so I booked a trip to Vermont. It hit home that one of the biggest things missing from my life in North Carolina was girlfriends.

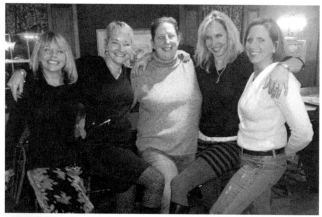

Williamstown gang—me with Cindy Lou Pou, Jane, and Mary

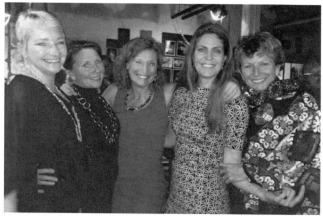

Me with Pink Ladies of Vermont—Terry, Andrea, Annette, and Lynn (Carol absent)

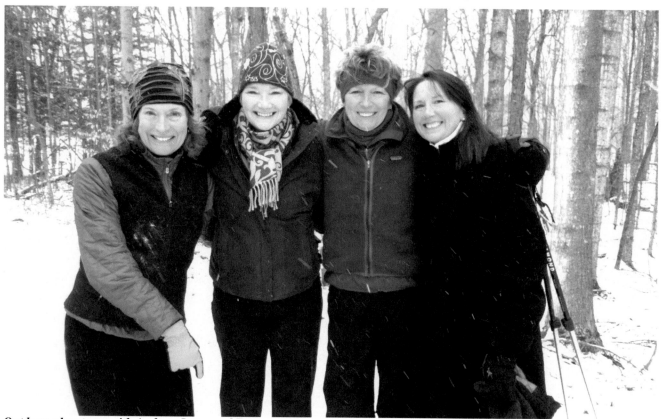

Outdoor adventures with Andrea, Lynn, and Terry

In my personal journal that I didn't share with anyone, I found these notes that I want to share because I didn't know how to take care of Cindy. I was having a hard time letting go of leaning on Craig.

So, what has changed for me . . . yes, I thought I never wanted to marry again after failing twice. Right now, I am not looking for marriage; I am looking for a partner to love and live life with. After going through a life-threatening disease, I realized that nothing else matters other than "true love." All I want is to "love deeply and fully" and to "live life to the fullest." Now I am questioning everything and all I know is that what I want is to "be in love and to live life." That is why I am so sad.

I am also sad because all I ever wanted since I was a little girl was to be a mom and a loving wife. For some reason I was not meant to have children. I am OK with that, but I do want to share my life with a partner and my best friend. I am a nurturing person and I have a lot of love to give. Maybe I scare others with this love . . . I don't know. Sometimes I feel like my love is wasting away being on my own . . . it's not fulfilling for me . . . it's lonely. I have to learn to take care of Cindy and to be honest with myself about what I want.

So where was I?? I decided to put on my oxygen mask and focus on Cindy and my healing, getting stronger, and getting involved in the community. I didn't have to decide about moving right now . . .

I decided to take another trip, and things got worse. I was already scheduled to go to Boston for the annual NEMOA conference. As president, I was responsible for leading this event for five hundred people. I decided to go to Maine before the Boston conference to ski—yes, to GET ON IT, and ski Black Hole and all the other double black diamond trails at Sunday River with my besties Fran and George. The trip north was awful. The flight was delayed. I had to drive from Portland to Bethel. I finally made it, ten hours after I left North Carolina.

Kim, Kathleen, and Kathleen's boys, Brant and Cole, were also up for the weekend, so we had a full house at George and Fran's Sunday River ski chalet. We had the best day skiing ever! Glorious spring skiing with bluebird skis and warm weather.

We always got out at 8 a.m. to be the first on the chair lift and we skied nonstop to get ten runs in by 10 a.m. for a hot chocolate break at North Peak. We typically left the mountain around noon or 1:00 to have paninis and beer back at the chalet.

This Saturday, March 9th, was no different. I was scared about skiing because of how weak I was from all the surgeries in 2012, but the Get REAL and HEEL program really helped me get stronger. I was not even close to pre-cancer Cindy, but I was strong enough to keep up with everyone. We skied Black Hole, the steepest double black on the mountain, and it was magnificent. We stood at the top and looked at one another and said, "GET ON IT! This is for Stu Dog!"

We were headed home at 1 p.m. for our paninis and beers. Fran, Kim, and George were in front of me, and Kathleen and her boys behind me, when the accident occurred.

Now back to my journal . . .

I NEED YOUR MOJO!

Written March 14, 2013 7:35 p.m. by Cindy Marshall

Hi Everyone,

Many of you know and some do not . . . so I am repeating the story and copying something I sent to my exercise friends . . .

I had the best day skiing last Saturday with my friends at Sunday River in Bethel, ME (Fran, George, Kathleen, Kim, and crew). We skied hard from 8 a.m. to 1:00 p.m. on gorgeous snowpack trails. It was the perfect spring skiing day with bright blue sunny skies and lots of hooting and hollering. I was sooooo happy and I felt strong on my skis. I even skied Black Hole, the steepest slope. GET ON IT!

On our way home, I was skiing on a flat by the main base lodge, Barker, and a snowboarder came flying down a connecting slope and collided with me. Yes, NOT good . . . he hit me hard. I was thrown into the air about five feet (according to one of my friend's sons who witnessed it) and did a complete flip and landed on my shoulder (twenty-five feet away). The ski patrol took care of me, picked me up, gave me oxygen and took me to the clinic in a

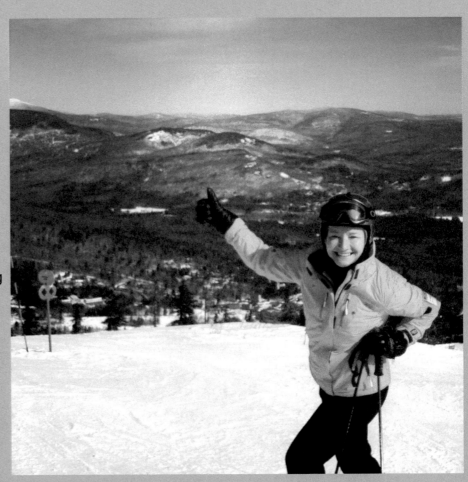

stretcher. Bottom line is that I broke my right shoulder—the humerus bone is broken off the humeral ball. It's completely broken off, very swollen and painful. I'm back on painkillers and will need surgery for a plate and screws to put me back together. I thought I was done with all this crap (but on the positive side, I didn't break my neck).

My breast surgeon from UNC, Dr. Amos, got me in to see the top orthopedic surgeon, Dr. Spang (NO, not Spanx but close . . . easy to remember). He is the orthopedic doctor for the UNC Tar Heel football and basketball teams! I have surgery tomorrow . . . 12 noon arrival at main hospital and then surgery at 2:30. I will be in hospital for at least one night but most likely two (per doctors' orders). I have a good friend here from Vermont, Terry Findeisen, and she is taking great care of me (THANK YOU TERRY!). Craig has been great as well and will be with me tomorrow and throughout the weekend (didn't expect any less from him, but it's a lot to deal with given all he had to deal with last year!).

I am grateful for everyone that is helping out . . . Mary, AOE, stepped in to shower me and do wash; Ed and Mary next door helped with airport runs; Andrea is coming down next week; Fran is shipping me her "designer slings and comfy clothes"; George drove my car to the airport; Fran, George, Kim, and Kathleen looked after me in Maine, others are helping out next week . . . thank you all!

Bad news: This will be a long recovery, six to nine months of physical therapy. Plus, it will be two to three weeks of rest before I can get back to work full time . . . ugh!! Good news: Bones heal and I have you for my love and support. Please send it all—feeling weak and down! Can't type any more . . .

Love and hugs,
Cindy

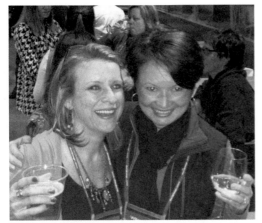

Laura and Linh

Sadly, I didn't make it to Boston for the NEMOA conference. I was so disappointed, because the NEMOA organization had been so supportive of me during my cancer treatments. They even decided to honor me with a NEMOA golf event during the summer. All funds raised went to cancer research. I was extremely grateful for the NEMOA board during this time, because they took over for me. Our VP of the board, Dana Pappas, used my talking points to present key points during the event. Dana even posted the picture of me in the orange jacket as part of the opening presentation. The NEMOA organization posted a flip chart for attendees to sign as a get-well card for me!! I was completely overwhelmed with love and gratitude. Several of my close friends that had worked for me over the years, and were now my mentees, sent me pictures of them toasting to me!

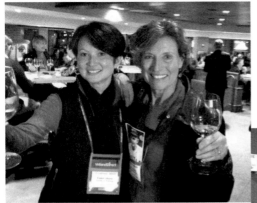

Linh and Andrea

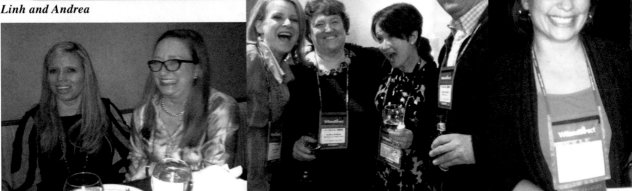

Stacey Hawes and Margot Murphy Moore, NEMOA board members

Laura, Ashley, Linh, and George

Terri Patasknik

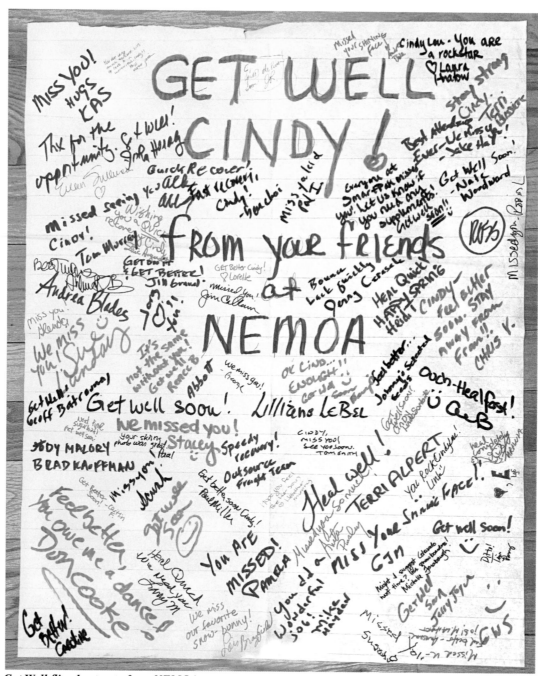

Get Well flip chart note from NEMOA

HOME, LOVE, BED, MEDS, AND ICE

Written March 19, 2013 9:21 a.m. by Cindy Marshall

Hi Everyone,

Yes, I'm home and in my own bed resting . . . yeah! Surgery went well and as the doctor wanted. He told me there was a chance they would need to do a bone graft as well as plates and screws. Good news—that wasn't needed! I finally got to my hospital room Friday night at 8:30 p.m. Craig and Terry were there to greet me when I woke and waited patiently until I was settled in my bed to leave. I ordered dinner at 9 p.m. and it arrived at 10 p.m., so I finally got food in my system after a long day.

The anesthesia team was there Friday night to put nerve blocker in. Thank God for that!! It helped so much. I was able to avoid the worst pain for the first two days and it allowed me to also avoid lots of narcotics like morphine! This allowed my head to be clear so I could sleep well! I made it through the hospital stay even though I had a bad roommate. The best part was my visitors!

Craig, my HMN (hot male nurse), is back in full swing . . . I feel so bad having to call on my HMN after all he did for me last year . . . but he has been willing, with that adorable smile, and for that I am extremely grateful!! Thank you, my handsome Craig, for all you do! First, he brought me lovely flowers, and he knows how to do flowers well! Then he showed up each morning at the hospital with my grande latte from Starbucks and a turkey bacon sandwich! Yum! Then he took Terry to Allen and Sons BBQ so she could experience the finest North Carolina BBQ. They showed up to visit me with my dinner of a pulled pork sandwich and cole slaw!! Wow, spoiled!! Craig was sporting his Wales rugby scarf proudly, as Wales beat England 30–3 in the rugby finals!!! Yahoo! Go Wales! He was also there on Sunday to take me home, and Poppy dog was home to greet me. I love you, Craig. Thank you for being there for me!! You are the best HMN!

Terry Findeisen, one of the Pink Ladies of Vermont, arrived Thursday to help me get ready. Thank you, Ed Owen, my fabulous neighbor, for collecting her at the airport! I am so grateful for Terry's visit! She helped me stock the house with food (of course she drove and lifted), bathed me, shaved my legs (feels good to be clean shaved), and fed me! Terry made sure I was delivered to the docs properly on Friday and she visited the hospital Saturday while I ate lunch. Then she went home and repaired my towel rack and other items in the house that needed TLC. She also kept Jag happy with food and love and kept Craig company! Wow, what a treat! Thank you, my dear friend Terry, for your love and tender care! You rock and I love you!

Mary, AOE, has also been amazing!! She came by several times last week to help me with laundry, changing the bed, washing me, shaving legs, getting mail, and taking tax prep to the accountant. Then she visited me at hospital Saturday bearing gifts! Then Mary came by Sunday afternoon to deliver lovely flowers from Vicky and Mary! Beautiful spring Easter assortment with tulips, iris, lilies, and hydrangea—I just love them—thank you Vicky for the thoughtful flowers and Mary for picking up and delivering! I love you both!

Then Cindy Lou Pou from Williamstown and her sister Lynn, who just moved to Raleigh, arrived Sunday afternoon for a brief visit. They brought a lovely violet plant and lots of cheerful smiles. It was so fun to have them here. I only wish I could have enjoyed more time with them and some wine together. Thank you both for visiting! Cindy is like a sister to me, and I loved having her here.

Shift two arrived on Monday . . . that would be Andrea Diehl, another Pink Lady of Vermont! Bill Calhoun picked her up at the airport, and they arrived mid-Monday with bags of ice. Andrea got me settled with my ice machine—my new best friend—and fed me lunch. Linh Calhoun arrived with dinner from Whole Foods, all sorts of goodies! Andrea will be here until Thursday, when neighbors take over. Thank you, Andrea and Linh. I love you both and appreciate you!

My left hand is tired of typing . . . Plus coffee is on its way . . . so another day is ahead and I'm grateful to be here living it. I just wish I didn't have to deal with the one-arm crap, but as Arletha, one of my nurses said, "Your time is not done, honey. God had more plans for you." So onward we go. GET ON IT!!

Heal quickly Whoville!

Thank you all for your love, prayers, and encouragement!
Love to all,
Cindy

WHOVILLE SAGA CONTINUES . . .

Written March 26, 2013 3:32 p.m. by Cindy Marshall

Hi All,

This will be short as I'm in pain and need a nap . . . but I wanted to share. Good news first: I saw ortho doc yesterday, and he said I was doing well. He took out most of the stitches but left in two or three that were not ready. He showed me the X-rays, which are exactly like Fran's from a year ago. It's a metal plate with nine screws . . . holy cow! Good news is that I know I will get through this, given the success I've seen with Fran. Bad news is that it will be a long journey of rehab. I start "at home PT" exercises twice a day for the next ten days, then start PT in Carrboro.

Bad, bad news: there is part of the IV catheter, about an inch, stuck in my left hand, and I now have surgery scheduled on Friday to take it out!! They did a bad job with the first IV. It kept snagging and finally broke off, so they redid it in my arm during the hospital stay. I am so mad about this . . . it's my good hand, the left one, so no idea what that means for recovery. It's outpatient and hopefully a local. Ughhhhhh.

One day at a time . . .
Keep prayers coming.
Love and hugs,
Whoville

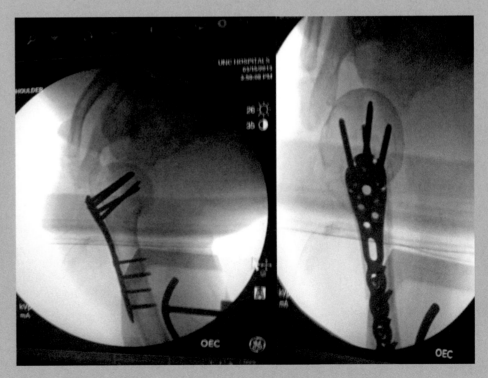

I withdrew my heart because I was feeling "LOVE RISK."

Chapter 20

A BROKEN HEART REFLECTION

I couldn't imagine life without Craig. I didn't know how to be alone, how to be Cindy and not to have a partner in life. However, in hindsight, this was the best thing that happened to me. I finally learned to take care of myself. I kept moving life forward and reached out to others to help me.

I withdrew my heart because I was feeling "love risk" and I didn't want Craig to have it anymore. Yes, I was vulnerable. What I didn't know was that I was still recuperating. I still had medicine and anesthesia in my body. I was alone. I was scared. I didn't know how to be the new me. On the business front, I was running SHINE Strategy and delivered great results. But on the personal front, I couldn't see how to move forward without Craig. I started visiting my parents in Asheville more frequently, which was a Godsend! I listened to them. I learned from them. I socialized with their friends. I became closer to them. I began to realize how grateful I was to have their genes and to be their daughter. It made me sad to think many people haven't experienced unconditional love from their parents. I know that some of my strength comes from my genes, but I also know that I learned how to be strong during my cancer phase. I always say to others, please love and care for yourself, so you don't have to get sick to figure it out the hard way, like I did!

Craig and I split up, and I was alone again. During this time, I reflected on everything I did wrong. Looking back on this, it was not healthy. The best thing I could have done was to look forward and feel grateful for each breath, but I still wasn't there yet. Someone once told me to be patient with life, that lessons will reveal themselves when you are ready to accept them. I was a very impatient person. I had no patience, so I didn't listen.

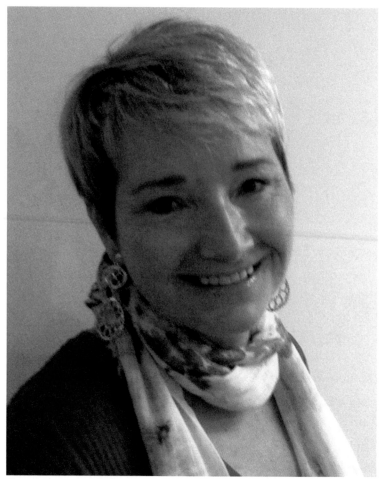
Sporting my new hair

My daily horoscope on April 7, 2013, was telling me to "loosen up," which of course is not easy for me! I always thought I could control the direction of my life, but I can't. Life happens, and I needed to accept what is next. I needed to float down the river and let my faith carry me on. I was in a constant state of reflection during this period. I reflected on my relationships with men. I was sad. I felt broken again. My heart was crushed.

Then I asked myself "What do I have?" I had my life. I finally realized how true the saying is: "You can't love someone else until you love yourself first." I started to listen to my inner voice. I started to listen to Cindy, to let go and live life. I found this story that I wrote to myself in my journal on April 13, 2013, and wanted to share it.

Craig swept me off my feet.

He taught me what it was like to be passionately in love and to care for another person. He helped me get through my divorce with a knowing that I was going to be OK.

I helped Craig feel love and joy again, I gave him happiness.

He taught me how to give and receive.

He was there for me every step of the way, through thick and thin. What happened? Was it all too much for him?

We were good for each other.

We shared a lot of great memories.

Every day, every step, everything I do, I think of Craig. UGH . . . I am having a hard time letting go.

I know it's not me . . . I know he loves me, and it hurts him too. Maybe I need to " truly be with Cindy and only Cindy."

Maybe I simply need this time to listen to my soul.

This just sucks and I am soooooo sad, but I know I can only give what one can handle! Right now, I think he has given me more than I can give but what can I learn from this?

What is the message?? What do I do? HEAL.

HAPPY GOOD FRIDAY!

Written March 29, 2013 4:12 p.m. by Cindy Marshall

Good Day Everyone!
Mine started early with a 5:45 a.m. pickup by Mary Sullivan, my AOE, to take me to UNC for surgery. This is my seventh surgery in a year, and I am claiming this to be the LAST one!

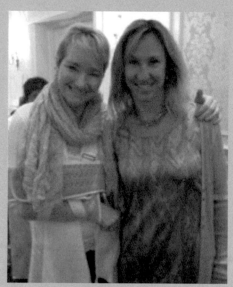

Me with Mary Edgerton

If you recall from my prior post, we thought there was part of an IV stuck in my hand from the shoulder surgery two weeks ago. Well, it turns out it was an inch-long blood clot! Good news: no catheter in me and they got it out, so I have less chance of having a blood clot traveling through my body!! Scary. Good news: I can still use my left hand! Bad news: I am drained from another surgery with strong meds, so resting today.

I want to wish you all a fabulous Easter weekend!! I will have a quiet weekend in Chapel Hill. I was planning to visit my folks in Asheville but can't drive, so hanging here. Craig is going on holiday to Hilton Head with his daughters, who are visiting from London, so I will see them tomorrow on their drive to the coast. Sunday, I will walk up the street to church, followed by brunch at the Duke Chapel with my good friend Mary Edgerton and her family.

I continue to be amazed by your love and support! I've received lots of cards and goodies—keep them coming! I've even been blessed with visits and help from many good friends: Terry F, Cindy Poulin and sister Lynn Gore, Andrea, Greg and Sandi Driscoll, Mary AOE, Mary and Ed Owen, Linh Calhoun, all my new Get REAL and HEEL (correct tar heel spelling) friends Vicky, Gail and Joan, and Mary Edgerton. And my dear beau Craig has been here as often as possible over the past few weeks. I feel blessed to have such care!

Also, thank you to everyone (near and far) for the chocolates, flowers, jellybeans, books, scarves, English treats, Easter bunny graham crackers, and a stuffed Eddy the Yeti from Sunday River (their mascot)!! Also, thank you Aunt Mary, my ninety-year young aunt, for the homemade Easter bunny and chicks!!! I love them and can't believe you made them for me!

Have a great Easter weekend and enjoy the NEW beginning!! I know I will. Onward and upward we go! I leave you with a quote from my daily read:

"The gift of shedding. From the beginning, the key to renewal has been the casting off of old skin . . . shedding opens us to self-transformation after transformation."

May you find newness as you cast off your dead skin and allow new transformations to begin!
Love to all!!
Cindy Lou Who, who is DONE with surgeries.

WHOOOO BEAR

Written April 5, 2013 6:20 p.m. by Cindy Marshall

Hi Everyone,
I wanted to share a few updates . . .

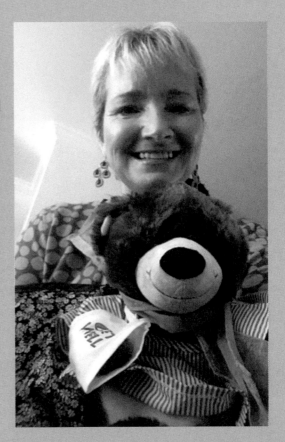

First update: I saw Dr. Spang (ortho) on Thursday, and he said I was doing really well, just where he expected me to be. Great news: I do not have to wear my sling when I am home, which helps me feel more normal, and I can try new things with the right hand. He also wants me to stop wearing the stabilizer (long strap piece) when I am out. So today I tested out a designer sling from Fran!!

In addition, Dr. Spang wants me to start doing motor skills like typing and cutting my food! How basic, but it is work . . . I am using my right hand now! One step at a time and one day at a time, I am learning to be patient. My only restriction is lifting; I can't lift anything heavier than a Coke can.

Second update: I had two PT appointments this week and I love my PT person, Smruti! She is wonderful. I made huge progress in two days. On Tuesday, we could barely get my arm to 45 degrees, and on Thursday we got it to 60! I also learned a few new exercises and I am working on continually rolling shoulders back and standing up straight, so I don't get frozen shoulder (when fluid in capsule around shoulder socket turns to gel and won't allow you to move).

Third update: I continue to be grateful for your love and support! I forgot to mention last time a few things people sent like new PJs and homemade cookies and vitamin C packets! THANKS!! This week I have gotten more goodies, and today I received "Whooo Bear" from Marilyn on the Vineyard. Marilyn, aka the Abbess, is one of my ski buddies from Sunday River, ME, and she suffered a terrible ski accident earlier this season and broke several bones in her leg. She had several surgeries and is slowly recuperating on the Vineyard. I sent her a get-well bear to cheer her up back in February; she has named the bear "Whooo," and here is the poem that came with Whooo, written by the Abbess herself:

Whooo Comes to Visit:

This year I found my calling
As I landed on the isle
To bring good cheer and happy smiles
To the injured for a while
The Abbess had been broken
While playing in the snow
How long she would be hobbling
Was very hard to know
She smiled and hugged me tightly
When she found me at her door
We fast became great buddies
Whooo couldn't ask for more
Not long after arriving
The snow snakes struck again
Snow boarders had collided
With our sender and good friend

Whoville became the victim
Of another broken bone
So it was clear my time on island
Would be ending sometime soon
So here I am dear Cindy
To bring you hugs so fast
I'll wear the ugly garments but
The scarf will help time pass
We will pass the time together
As your shoulder mends and heals
I am here to make you happy
For I know how you must feel
Just set me on the sofa
Look at me and know
It is only time that is passing
For we have far to gooooooo~~~~~~

HOW AWESOME IS THAT??!!

I love you, Abbess, and thank you for the gift of Whooo!!

I am happy as I heal surrounded by all your love! Thank you everyone for your kindness and good cheer! Keep it coming—I need it!!

With love and WHOOO hugs,
Whoville and Whooo Bear

SHAVING LEGS
Written April 7, 2013 9:34 p.m. by Cindy Marshall

YAHOOOOO! I successfully shaved my legs today all by myself!! That's progress—yeah!! I have to say that I wasn't really happy when the hair on my legs grew back from chemo because I loved NOT having to shave, but now it grows like crazy. Yes, I am counting my blessings and I am thankful that my hair is growing!!!

I do want to thank the five ladies that helped me get through the last three weeks of leg shaving. First, Mary Sullivan, my AOE, who was very cautious and slow—maybe left a few hairs behind—but we were thrilled just to have legs shaved! Second, Terry Findeisen, who I playfully called the aggressive leg shaver, but she did a great job! Third Andrea Diehl, who wanted to make sure she shaved in a straight line . . . ha! We giggled over that. Fourth, my Get REAL and HEEL friend Vicky Bryant, who was careful and calm. And last but not least, Linh Calhoun, who was the shy one—she was scared at first and afraid of cutting my leg—but then got the hang of it and did a great job!! Everyone was fabulous and I am so grateful for their help!! I'm happy to say you ladies are now successfully off the hook of "leg shaving duty."

I continue to get stronger daily . . . today I stopped meds during the day, but now I am ready for bed and need some. One day at a time . . . Whoville will be back and stronger than before!

Thanks again for all your love and support!!
Love,
Whoville

GRATEFUL FOR TODAY!

Written April 17, 2013 10:04 p.m. by Cindy Marshall

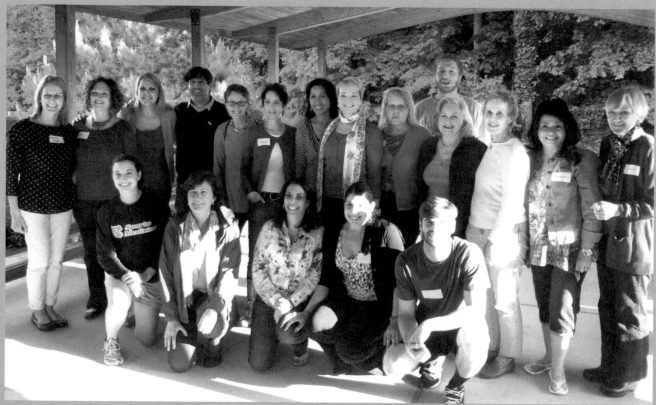

Get Real and Heel Team at UNC

I've been having a tough time lately, for many reasons, but today I regained some strength! YEAH!!

I went to my 8 a.m. Get REAL and HEEL post–breast cancer care class at UNC (sponsored by Susan G. Komen) and walked away grateful to have been there and to be involved with such fabulous ladies! It was just what I needed today. I was able to ride the incumbent bike, walk the tennis court loop, and do lunges and ab work! Yahoo! This made me feel normal again. You may recall that I started this program in January and was halfway through when my I broke my arm/shoulder.

Exercise was followed by a social gathering with the five women from my group and five others from another group. We learned breathing and relaxation techniques. First, we learned how to do a complete body scan, which is a transcendental meditation technique that totally relaxes your body and mind. The mantra we repeated in our head as we were guided through the process was, "Everything will be OK; you are exactly where you are supposed to be." It was very moving! We also learned the "bellows breath technique" designed to wake you up and give you energy. It works great, and there are many videos online about it. The last technique was called "relaxation breathing 4–7–8" which teaches you to breathe in for four seconds, hold for seven, and exhale for eight. It sounds simple, but it takes concentration, especially because your tongue has to be in a certain position on the roof of your mouth. Bottom line, they were all useful and very good discussions were had among all of us.

I am so grateful to have been given the opportunity to be part of Get REAL and HEEL. It's been just what I needed to help with closure on breast cancer and to move on. I only wish every cancer patient was lucky enough to experience this. My sister-in-law Barbara told me about a class she went to in Cleveland yesterday that helped her. She shared a quote about courage with me that I want to pass on:

"Courage does not always roar. Sometimes courage is the quiet voice at the end of the day saying I will try again tomorrow."

I send all of you courage to get on with the next challenge in your life, and to everyone in Boston for the tragedy of Monday's senseless and awful event at the Boston Marathon, GET ON IT—have courage—it will be OK!

I am also grateful for all of you and thank you again for caring about Whoville as I work on putting my body back together yet once again. But rest assured, my spirit will never fail and will always be strong and positive!!

Love,
Whoville

(aka Humpty Dumpty, who fell down but got back up again and carried on!)

ONE YEAR POST CHEMO AND TATTOOS . . .

Written April 29, 2013 8:13 p.m. by Cindy Marshall

Hi All,

This past Thursday, April 25th, I was visiting with girlfriends Leann, Stefanie, and Joan in Concord, MA. When our waiter asked what we were celebrating, we looked at each other and said GIRLFRIENDS!! Yes, that is true—girlfriends are the secret sauce to life! But that night when I woke up at 3 a.m. for the usual hot flash, I realized it was the anniversary of my LAST chemo at UNC and that is something to celebrate!!! Yahoo!! That also means it's one more month until I hit my one-year cancer FREE mark! Another big celebration!

I had a great weekend in Boston—quality time with Leann and Paul in Concord, then girls' night out at 80 Thoreau on Thursday. It was great to see my "big sishta" Joan Litle and spend some quality time at dinner. Friday, I saw some of my fabulous NEMOA pals in Boston for our board meeting. It was so great to see them, especially because I missed the big spring event in Boston due to my shoulder break.

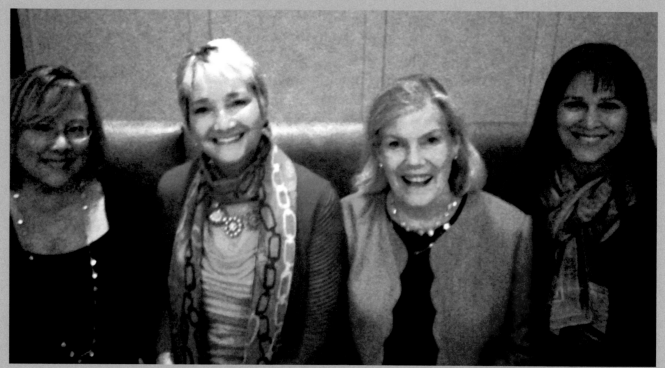

Me with Leann, Joan, and Stefanie

Friday night, I met up with Maura Maloney, my good girlfriend from college and a breast cancer survivor! We had a ball—lots of giggling and girl time. I left Maura's midday Saturday to drive to Acton, MA, to spend the next twenty-four hours with Rob and Stefanie Jandl, my good friends from Williamstown, and two of their children, Luke and Elise. We relaxed, talked, had a fabulous dinner, and drank some awesome wine! Stefanie and I had lots of girl time, which was rejuvenating! Girlfriends are the best!!

When I flew home to Chapel Hill Sunday afternoon, I learned that my steel plate sets off the TSA alarms and requires a FULL pat down that takes fifteen minutes . . . they touched everything!! Now I know how to plan my travel.

This morning at 8:30, I was picked up by Zully Blake to take me to UNC for my nipple tattoos! HA! Yes, I now have two tattoos—wild! It was more painful than I thought, and we are not done yet; I still have one or two more visits. We cracked up when my fabulous nurse, Sue Hayden, brought out trays of colors to choose from. We tried on several colors and selected what we liked best—the most natural, of course. We then had to select the right size areola—even more funny! I am bandaged up right now and will not know the full effect until my shower tomorrow . . . something to look forward to!

So onward we go. My shoulder is healing slowly; some days are worse than others. One day at a time . . . I continue to be grateful for every breath and for my circle of LOVE—all of YOU! Thank you!!

Love,
Whoville

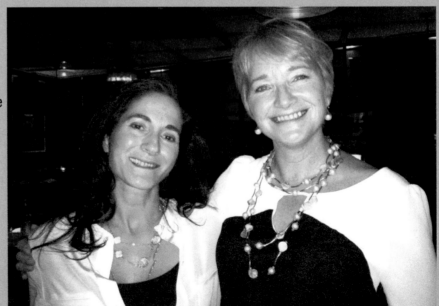
Me with Maura

I will always be grateful for
this LOVE of FRIENDSHIP,
COMPASSION, and ADMIRATION.

Chapter 21

GRATEFUL GETAWAY

One of my very good friends from the catalog industry, Lois Brayfield, gifted me the use of her spectacular home on the island of St. John for a vacation to recuperate. Lois and I had known each other for years as leaders in the catalog industry. We both served on the Direct Marketing Association catalog conference committees. I asked Lois to join me on the board of directors at NEMOA because we needed her brilliant and creative mind. It was during this time that I learned about Lois's gracious, caring, and loving soul. She was by my side during my illness and supported me deeply with her love and spiritual prayers. I will always be grateful for her love of friendship, compassion, and admiration.

Craig and I were scheduled to go on this vacation to St. John in mid-May, but we both decided it wasn't the right thing to do given our time apart. I decided to ask one of my best friends, Daria, who lives in Ireland but was coming to America to spend time with her family. We had a spectacular time together, giggling the entire time and exploring the island together. I had only been to St. John on a sailboat with my second husband but never stayed long enough to explore the island. Daria and I tried new restaurants, found hidden beaches, searched for seashells, ate ice cream, shopped, and had loads of girlfriend time talking about life. It was just what I needed to begin to heal and remember who Cindy was as I approached one year cancer free.

When I returned from St. John, I went to my parents' house for Memorial Day weekend. On the way to my parents' in Asheville, I drove by the Audi dealer just miles from their home, and I saw it—my dream car. Yes, a black Audi Cabriolet convertible for sale! The next day, which happened to be the Saturday of Memorial Day weekend, I told my parents I had an errand to run. I headed to the dealer and checked out the Cabriolet. I showed them my Passat wagon, and they gave me a price for the trade-in. We negotiated and I bought the car!!

Holy COW! What have I done? It will be cleaned and ready for pick up on Monday, Memorial Day. This was such a crazy feeling . . . but I felt alive and excited for each new day. I loved the "wind in my hair" feeling and the warm sunshine on my face. This convertible was a symbol of freedom to me. I named her Whoville Freedom, and of course my North Carolina plate was Whoville, so it was perfect! I loved my Whoville convertible; we spent a lot of happy and sad times together.

EIGHTEEN MONTHS . . .

Written May 22, 2013 10:58 p.m. by Cindy Marshall

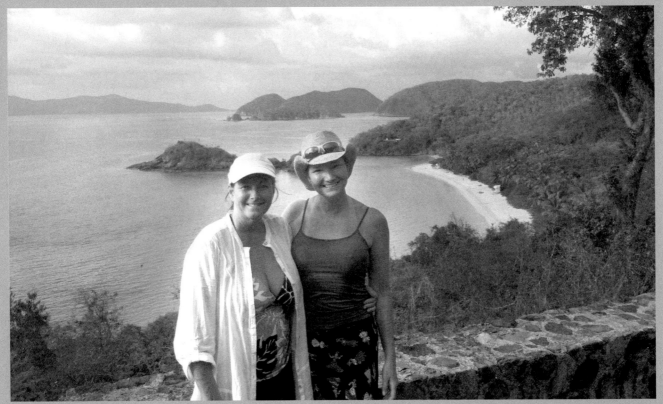

Me with Daria, St. John

Hi Everyone,

I got the urge to write this journal today because of a conversation I had last night while chatting with Vicky. Vicky reminded me that today would mark the eighteen-month anniversary of the passing of Stu Jones, her beloved husband. Stu was not only a great father to Fran and Sarah, but a fabulous father-in-law to George (except when he beat George at golf) and a great friend to all—Mary, Marilyn, Peter, Mabel, Ruthie, Joanne, Terrie Ann, and many others, including me!

I know the last eighteen months have not been easy for Vicky, Fran, George, and Sarah, but I also know that Stu Dog, our affectionate canary, has also been there to watch over all of us and help us carry on, no matter

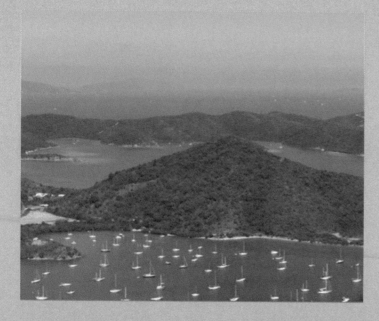

what. Stu was like a second father to me, and I am grateful to have known him and to have been part of his life.

It was at Stu's funeral service that I decided to get the pain in my left breast checked out (thank you Stu, Shawn, Debbie, Liz, and Kim for encouraging me). I was diagnosed with breast cancer just five days after his service, and my eighteen-month journey began . . .

For many of you, eighteen months may seem like a short period of time, but the last eighteen months for me were LONG, hard, painful, emotional, scary, and very beautiful. I also know it was a long, hard time for my family, for Craig, and for all of you, my circle of love. But we did it—we GOT ON IT and we survived this eighteen-month journey.

I am a better person for having experienced the last eighteen months. I learned a great deal and will share my learnings with you when I complete my book. One thing was very clear to me: YOUR support and love was abundant, and you helped me get through this tough time. For that I am very grateful. THANK YOU!

The photo is Daria and me on St. John's a week ago, totally relaxed and in island mode . . .

Love to all,
Cindy, aka Whoville

The next week marked the one-year anniversary of my bilateral mastectomy on May 30th. This was the day I considered myself "cancer free" because it was when all my cancer was removed. It was when Dr. Amos told me, "You are a complete pathological response!" meaning I followed the textbook path of treatment. The chemo did its job and killed the cancer inside me. On May 30th I was invited to visit the corporate offices of Extended Stay America, which would later become a SHINE Strategy client.

During my time as president of Exclusively Weddings, I met some incredibly talented young leaders. One of them was Christopher Thomas-Moore, affectionately known at CTM. CTM was a project leader, marketing mastermind, and business driver whom I mentored. He became a trusted resource for me at Exclusively Weddings and was instrumental in the launch of Exclusively Gifts, a personalized gift business. This was the second time I had my photo on page two of a catalog, which was an honor.

When we were building Exclusively Gifts, we needed a great writer for content, so we hired Andrea Diehl, whom I worked with at the Vermont Country Store. Andrea was brilliant! Andrea, as you know from my journal earlier, became one of my best friends and was part of "the pink ladies of Vermont" and an amazing caretaker of mine. My team at Exclusively Weddings loved working with her!

CTM moved on to be the Senior Director of Ecommerce and Digital Marketing at Extended Stay America, which eventually became a SHINE Strategy client. CTM was extremely supportive of me while I was sick. He knew my one-year cancer free anniversary was coming up on May 30th, so he organized a celebratory dinner with several former colleagues and friends of mine. CTM invited Andrea, Megan, and Ali to join us. Andrea was in town from Vermont working on some copy projects. Megan Karney, a former Exclusively Weddings marketing analyst, was working for CTM as his Senior Manager of Digital Marketing at Extended Stay. And Ali McGraw, former product manager of Exclusively Weddings, who was now at Belk, joined us. It was such a treat to visit Extended Stay to see CTM shine in his new Director role. I also loved seeing Andrea succeed in her consulting role, as well as connecting with Megan and Ali, who were advancing in their careers and becoming very successful.

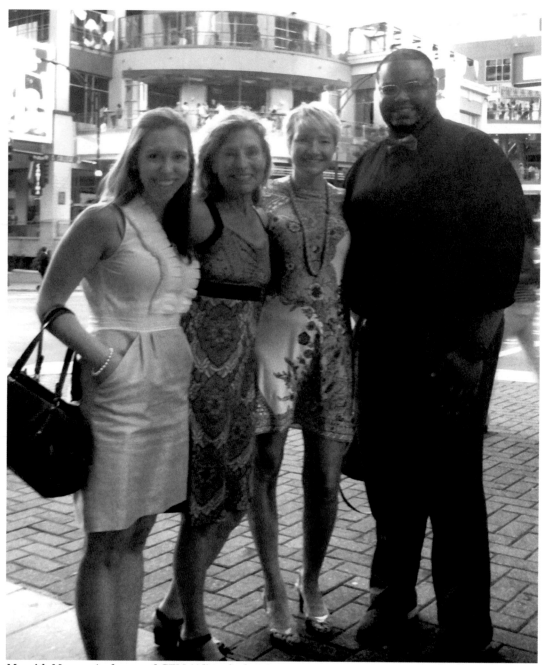

Me with Megan, Andrea, and CTM (Ali took photo)

Collectively, they gave me a special celebratory card with a picture of a chocolate chip cookie:

Tough Cookie (tuhf kook-e)–noun

1. Someone with just the right mix sweetness and strength.
2. One who doesn't crumble under pressure.
3. A fighter who's too busy kicking butt to sit down and cry but knows it's OK to do both.
4. A person who doesn't always ask for support but has lots of friends who would do anything to help.

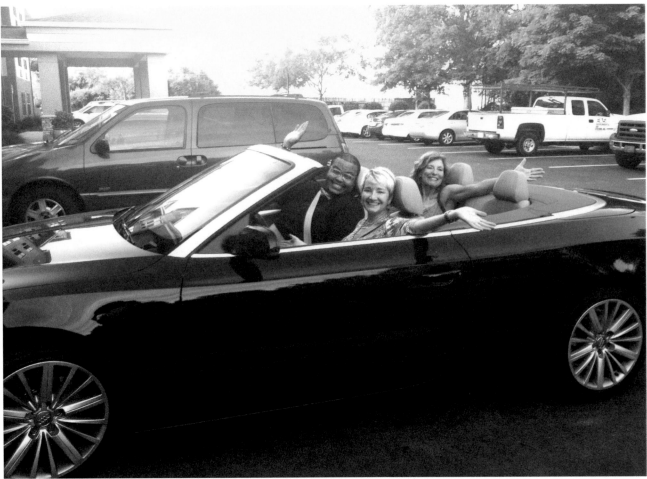

Me with CTM and Andrea in Freedom

Get REAL and HEEL

Chapter 22

ANOTHER ANGEL EARNS THEIR WINGS

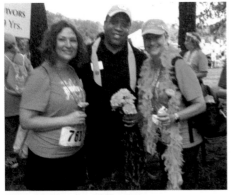

Me with Traci and Dr. Amos

June was full of deep emotions. The month started out joyful for me because I was celebrating being a one-year cancer survivor. I participated in the UNC Get REAL and HEEL walk on June 8th and ran into a lot of my UNC friends as well as Dr. Keith Amos, my breast surgeon. Dr. Amos and his girls were handing out roses to patients and survivors as we lined up for our processional. They asked us to stand in line based on our survival status, and I made it by one week to stand with the one-year survivors! I was beyond joyful and grateful!

Deep sadness set in mid-month when we learned that Dr. Amos died unexpectedly at the age of forty-two on June 18th from a brain aneurysm upon arrival in Edinburgh, Scotland. He had been so excited about his trip, and my heart went out to his wife and three young daughters, who were with him. He was a gentle, ever-so-calm, and reassuring presence. He was friends with all his patients, especially me, who relied on him in so many ways. The world lost a great one. His memorial service was at the end of the month on June 29th, and was standing room only. Craig and I cried together while we remembered Dr. Amos. I believe his story is best told by the experts at UNC and a few meaningful posts on his remembrance website.

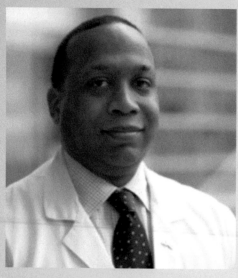

June 18, 2013 Announcement from UNC School of Medicine
Dr. Keith Amos Remembered
Caring doctor, avid researcher, engaged collaborator and effective teacher

UNC has lost a dear colleague. Dr. Keith Amos died suddenly in Edinburgh, Scotland, while on a Dr. Claude Organ, Jr., Travel Award from the American College of Surgeons. We all hold in our thoughts his wife, Ahaji, and their three young daughters.

Dr. Amos was a treasured member of the UNC School of Medicine, the Department of Surgery, the Division of Surgical Oncology, and the UNC Lineberger Comprehensive Cancer Center. He was a caring doctor, avid researcher, engaged collaborator, effective teacher and just a terrific human being. Colleagues, medical students, surgery residents and especially patients, to whom he was so dedicated, will sorely miss him.

Dr. Amos was passionate about visiting communities to talk about cancer, the importance of cancer screening, and cancer disparities. He traveled across North Carolina collaborating with and speaking to numerous groups, who always appreciated and were impressed by his commitment and dedication. He was a true ambassador for the University of North Carolina.

Dr. Amos was recruited to UNC in 2007. He earned his medical degree from Harvard University and completed surgery residency at Washington University in Saint Louis. His passion for cancer education and care led him to a Surgical Oncology fellowship at the M.D. Anderson Cancer Center in Houston.

While interviewing for his faculty position, he read the plaque located in the lobby of N.C. Memorial Hospital that states, "Operated for and by the People of North Carolina." He frequently said, "I think that's a really powerful statement. One of the things that attracted me here is that UNC is a state institution. We as physicians have an obligation to care for and educate citizens about their health problems."

Dr. Amos honored that commitment, and during his short career at UNC, focused his significant energy on all aspects of the multidisciplinary UNC Breast Center in Chapel Hill, Raleigh and across the state.

Cindy Marshall
Posted June 20, 2013 at 4:41 p.m.

I am still so devastated and at a loss for words . . . but I finally found some . . . Dr. Amos was my HERO, and he saved my life! Not only was he a FABULOUS doctor, but he was also a great friend to me and my family. His family was his life and I know how much he loved them—he would light up when he talked about them. My heart aches for his lovely wife and three young girls. So sad and so unfair. I had the pleasure of meeting his family for a brunch in Charlotte before the Cowboys vs. Panthers game. Of course, you all know what a diehard Cowboys fan Dr. Amos was—it was such a treat to share that time with him and to see him outside of the hospital.

Dr. Amos helped guide me through my treatment plan when I was diagnosed with aggressive triple negative breast cancer. It was under his love and care, along with many other fabulous doctors and nurses at UNC, that I beat cancer in just six months. When I had my check-up after my bilateral mastectomy in May of 2012, Dr. Amos gave me the biggest hug and said, "You are a complete pathological response!" Which meant that the chemo worked—it killed my 5 cm of tumors in my left breast and there was no sign of any cancer left! YAHOO!!

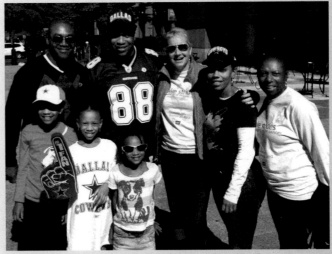

Me with Dr. Amos, his family, Heather, and Mark

Dr. Amos was the one who coached me through every step, and I saw him just one week before he left on his trip to the UK at the Race for the Cure—he gave me a carnation and so did his youngest girl! That is how I will always remember Dr. Amos, my HERO, doing what he loved—making others happy! I love you Dr. Amos and will miss you terribly!!! Thank you for giving me my life. I am just so sorry and sick to my stomach that you were taken away so soon . . . not fair. My love, prayers, strength, and sympathy goes out to Ahaji and the girls!!!

Eric Halvorson (my plastic surgeon)
Posted June 21, 2013 at 8:45 a.m.

Keith was always smiling and reading all these comments tells me why: he was always doing what he loved, following his heart, and I think the good he did in the world reflected in him this way. As a plastic surgeon specializing in cancer reconstruction, I worked very closely with Keith for 5 years, the entire time we both worked at UNC. In Keith I found a true colleague—I am grateful to have had the opportunity to work with him. His patients loved him dearly and his compassion was infectious and genuine. I cannot describe his good doctoring better than his patients have here, but I do want to add that he was also a technically SUPERB surgeon. He had it all, and he gave it all. He cared deeply about treating cancer, but he also made sure to do whatever he could to improve their reconstruction. There is a headlamp in the UNC operating room with Cowboys stickers and "Famous Amos" written on it. It always made me smile to see him operating with that. So few are capable of what he did—excellent surgeon, caring doctor, university ambassador, advocate for the underserved, sophisticated researcher, inspiring teacher and mentor, kind and warm human being, family man. He will always inspire us to be better doctors. I will miss you friend, and I'll always hear you chuckling and saying "that's right, that's right" after a good joke. To his girls—you were his light and now he will be yours.

Amy DePue (one of my nurses)
Posted June 23, 2013 at 9:27 p.m.

I believe with all my heart that knowing Keith Amos was a blessing in my life. Learning from him and getting to work with him were bonus blessings as well. May we continue to strive to serve breast cancer patients as thoughtfully as he did. My heartfelt condolences to his family. He is missed.

Traci Lloyd (Get REAL and HEEL friend)
Posted June 29, 2013 at 10:26 a.m.

My heart is broken. The world has lost a bright light in the passing of Dr. Keith Amos. Dr. Amos was my surgeon for 2 procedures in May and June of 2012. He also called me at 9:00 at night with pathology results so I wouldn't have to go to bed one more night without knowing. I had complications after my second surgery, and he spent time with me on the phone on a Sunday morning taking care of me. During the course of my treatment, there was a debate over what path to take. Dr. Amos interceded and spent time with me (along with Dr. Muss) to make sure that I was comfortable with my treatment plan. Dr. Amos told me, "I am not only your surgeon, I am your advocate." I have never seen anyone with such passion and dedication to their patients. He made you feel as if you were his only patient. The qualities that made him such a unique and wonderful physician are not learned; they were a part of his soul. Dr. Amos was a central figure in my cancer treatment and survival. I feel very lost without him, as I am sure many other patients do as well. He truly had a profound effect on my life. I am deeply saddened to know that there will be many future patients that will not experience his care. But the greatest loss is his role as a husband and father. My heart aches for his wife and daughters. I am continuing to lift you up in prayer. His daughters have a great legacy of caring, compassion, and dedication to carry on. I look forward to seeing the great women they will become.

Craig Waller (my loving partner)
Posted June 30, 2013 at 10:37 a.m.

I met Dr. Amos as he was guiding my partner, Cindy Marshall, through the frightening and bewildering path of breast cancer treatment and surgery. I was able to witness the incredible personal attention and commitment that so many people have talked about in their posts as he lavished it on Cindy. He became a guide and a mentor to her, and she would always defer a decision on each stage of her treatment until we learned "what Dr. Amos thinks."

As someone who has spent his life in business and with thankfully little exposure to the medical community, I was blown away by the humanity and compassion that all the staff of the Oncology unit—and especially Dr. Amos—showed at all times. You are an amazing group of people and, as I sat in the Memorial Service yesterday, I realized that I didn't know the half of what Keith Amos brought to the world and those that he touched in such a short life.

We were talking one day during Cindy's treatment, and he mentioned that he was going to Baltimore for a conference and staying at The Four Seasons Hotel. That happened to be an easy favor that I could do for him, to thank him for all he was doing for us, so (with me being under the mistaken impression that he was taking his wife with him) I arranged for his room to be upgraded and some wine and fruit to be sent to the room. When I saw him later, he thanked me for the room upgrade. "What did you like best about it," I asked, "the room itself, the view, the service?" He paused for a second. "The best part of it was that I was on the same floor as the President of the Association," he smiled, "and he couldn't figure out how I had got the same level room as him!"

From all the remembrances of yesterday this exchange resonated in retrospect and the famous Amos competitive streak had been revealed to me!

He was a man who made a huge impression on me in a very short time, and I've been deeply affected by his passing. My love goes to Ahaji and his girls—he was a great man, and clearly a loving husband and a wonderful father. The world is a far poorer place without him.

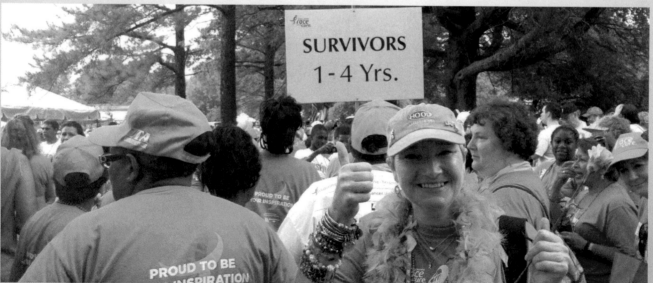

From all the remembrances
of yesterday this exchange
resonated in retrospect
and the famous Amos
competitive streak had been
revealed to me!

This was my time.
This was time to focus
on Cindy, on healing,
on writing, and on building my
SHINE Strategy business.

Chapter 23

ADVENTURES ON THE ROAD

My world in North Carolina was not well glued, and I felt the need to get away. I was loving my new Audi Cabriolet convertible; I called her Freedom. I felt alive when I was driving her "topless," yes—with the top down! I felt light and sunshine warming me with love. I was ready for a road trip. I also wanted to write my book, so I reached out to my good friends Sid and Curtis, who live in NYC and Vermont, and asked them if I could stay at their Vermont condo for the month of July to write my book. They were so gracious and said, "Absolutely, be our guest!" This was transformational!!

This was my time. This was time to focus on Cindy, on healing, on writing, and on building my SHINE Strategy business. I also knew that Craig needed time alone to build his life. We had taken a pause from each other to focus on ourselves and we were no longer dating, so I didn't feel the need to stay in North Carolina. I had very few friends in Chapel Hill, and I was longing for my Vermont girlfriends!

Daria, one of my best friends, sent me a meaningful poem on June 27, 2013, while I was getting ready for my five weeks in Vermont. It was just what I needed. *Let it go and be free in your new car Freedom, wind in the hair! Let it all go and begin again!* The poem was about letting go of the ways I thought life would unfold. To stop holding on to the plans, dreams, or expectations I had. Let it all go! All these messages were coming from the universe to me and I was finally learning to listen to them. I needed to let go and find the place of rest and peace from this transformation of life.

I left for Vermont on July 2nd, and the drive was so powerful. I was an emotional roller coaster again. My daily horoscope was on the mark!! It was all about changing—my life had been one massive change for the last eighteen months and now I was about to blossom into a shiny sunflower. Someone once told me, "If it doesn't challenge you, it doesn't change you." I was clearly a very different person. I was challenged. I was changed.

Again, my horoscope was sending me messages: "Establishing your own rhythm is healthier than attempting to conform to someone else's expectations." This is what I need to hear, because I needed to establish my rhythm and focus on Cindy.

I remember how the drive made me feel. I was free, I was on my own, I was in control of my life, I was so excited to reunite with my Vermont friends, and I was relieved I had a focus—my health and my book. I wrote down some of my thoughts during the drive when I stopped for breaks.

- *EXPECTATIONS – Don't have high expectations; let it be and relax.*

- *LIVE – Live life to the fullest, take it all in, stop and smell the flowers, be present.*

- *FREEDOM – The sense of letting my life in North Carolina go. I am free, I am in control of me and my business. I have no debt. I am building SHINE.*

- *FIREFLIES AND LIGHTNING BUGS – I loved fireflies as a child. They represented summer and were always around us shining their light. Craig called them lightning bugs and we used to watch them light up his back yard and smile with delight. I reflected on the difference between fireflies and lightning bugs and decided lightning bugs should be their name because they light up the sky and share their light with others. That is what I want to do—SHINE brightly for all to see.*

- *SOON YOUR TIME WILL COME – I keep getting messages from my inner voice to have patience, that soon my time will come. Maybe this is God talking or angels in heaven like Aunt Emmy, Aunt Nancy, or Aunt Mary, but the message is strong.*

- *LOVE, FAMILY, AND FRIENDS – Nothing else matters in life other than LOVE, FAMILY, and FRIENDS. You can take LOVE with you when you die, but not your possessions.*

- *"DREAMS" BY FLEETWOOD MAC – This song is very meaningful to me, and the lyrics struck a chord deep down—it is my song for this period of my life! It helps me remember what I have and what I lost. It helps me think about being free to choose waking up happy, not sad. Even though I lost a part of me, I still have my organs and body that function, even with a broken shoulder. It's time to live life and stop being sad about what I don't have and start being grateful for what I do have!*

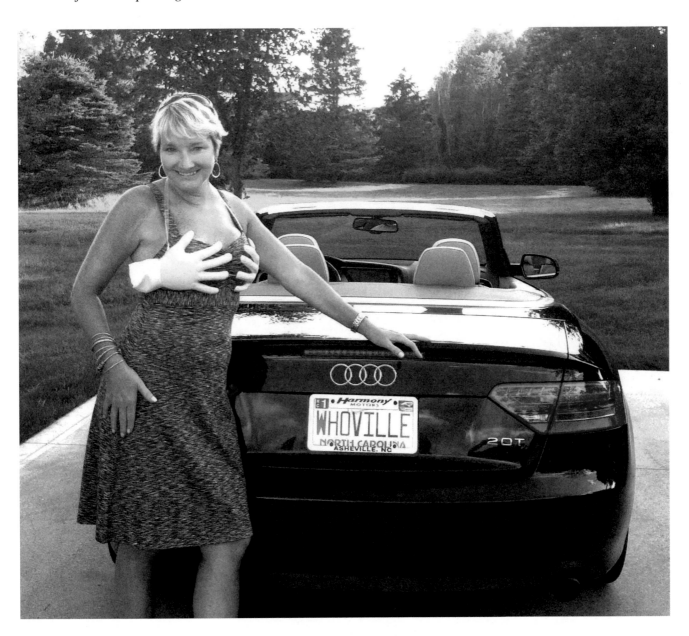

I have always thought there was a vortex in Manchester that is filled with magic—I surely felt it.

Chapter 24

VERMONT, A SUNFLOWER REBIRTH

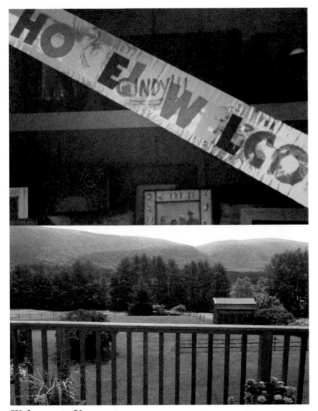

Welcome to Vermont

I arrived in Manchester, VT, and was welcomed with a massive love from Sid and Curtis. They decorated their home with "welcome home" banners, balloons, and flowers. I have always thought there was a vortex in Manchester that was filled with magic—I surely felt it. Manchester is in the valley of the Green Mountains of southern Vermont, and it truly is a magical place.

My right arm was no longer in a sling from my shoulder surgery, but it was only at 50% range of motion, so Curtis suggested we go to restorative hot yoga. The class was Friday mornings, so off we went on day two to hot yoga. This was truly the beginning of my transformation. I couldn't do all the poses and had to use a chair for some of them, but the teacher, Gianna Rose, was extremely helpful in guiding me. After the first class, we started talking and I learned that Gianna was also a skilled masseuse and had worked on breast cancer patients before. We decided to take her class each Friday and I would stay for a massage afterwards. I was thrilled and I could tell that the hot yoga was great for opening my shoulder muscles.

The first weekend in Manchester, Sid and Curtis threw me a "pink" party with about thirty of my close friends. I was completely blown away and I felt so loved. It was so nice to be with all my Vermont friends telling stories, giggling, and enjoying life. All of them had been so supportive of me over the past eighteen months, but they did it from Vermont while I was in North Carolina, so it was extra special to be together in person.

During the weekdays, I would write down thoughts for my book and do some SHINE work. I ended up getting busier with SHINE than I expected, because I signed new brands Orvis and Brooks Brothers. It was great to be busy with work, but this meant I couldn't do as much writing as I was hoping. There were lessons in patience and letting life happen versus planning it.

My Fridays were extremely magical. Curtis and I did the hot yoga, then I had my massage with Gianna. What I didn't know was that Gianna was a medium. The first massage, she said to me, "Why are you keeping your crown chakra closed?" I had no idea I was; maybe I was still in protection mode. She told me the room was filled with spirits for me. They were all around, and they wanted me to open my crown to listen to them. She said there was a woman with amber eyes who was there. I felt it was my Aunt Emmie, my mother's oldest sister who passed away at eighty-nine in 2011, just before I was diagnosed. I was very close to Aunt Emmie, who was also very close to my mother. We had a special bond. Aunt Emmie was sixteen years old when my mother was born and she helped raise my mother. I will never forget my last phone call with Aunt Emmie before she died. She called to ask me to "take care of her Janie and make sure she was OK." I promised I would, because I knew my mother had started going through memory loss and old-age dementia the year Emmie died.

After that, I began to listen to the messages being sent to me. During my weekly massages, Gianna would share new messages with me, and more spirits would be in the room. I realized that during my sickness, I had shut down my intuition and my ability to hear messages from the universe and angels around us. This was transformational for me. I began to be myself and to be more open. I explored other

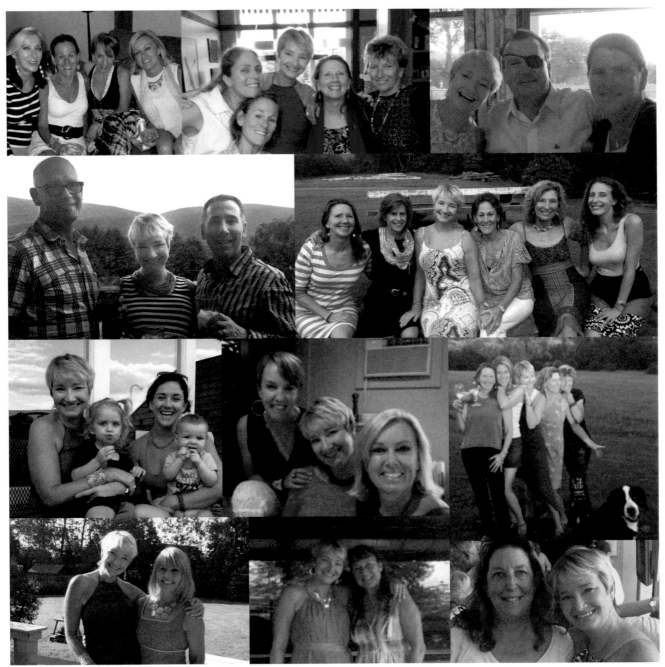

A collage of photos from the five weeks in Vermont that transformed my life

parts of Vermont and reconnected with my former sister-in-law Renee from Stowe. I explored, listened, played, learned, laughed, relaxed, and lived life.

At the end of the five weeks, Sid and Curtis threw me another party to send me back to North Carolina. All my friends came, and during this event, Sid made a toast that said, "Cindy's light is back. She was a wilted sunflower when she arrived five weeks ago, but now she is glowing and shining bright." That July was my sunflower rebirth. I was grateful for all my friends and for having the opportunity to experience my rebirth and ability to SHINE.

During those five weeks, I became more confident and trusting in myself. I was at peace with life and not afraid of the future. I felt closer to God and the angels around us. I felt confident in my ability to take charge of my life and control my own destiny. I believe that we control the small steps in life and God controls the bigger plans in life, like living five minutes from the UNC Chapel Hill cancer center.

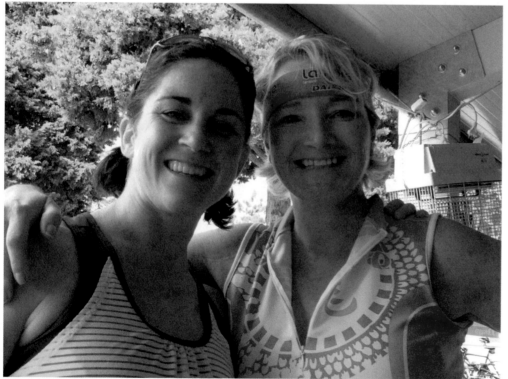

I went back to North Carolina after the five weeks in Vermont and then decided to move back to Vermont that October and never left. I even did a hypnotic regression in 2014 that told me I was exactly where I was supposed to be, in Vermont.

Me and Gianna Rose

I became more confident and trusting in myself. I was at peace with life and not afraid of the future.

I was meant to be living in Vermont and not North Carolina.

Chapter 25

REUNITED

When I got back to North Carolina in August, Craig had organized a romantic getaway to the mountains in Asheville for a fly fishing adventure. It was a magical weekend, and we were glowing spending time together. We continued to live our separate lives in our respective homes and talked frequently. I ended up traveling back to Vermont at the end of August for business with Orvis. While there, I realized I missed it so much and that I was meant to be living in Vermont and not North Carolina, so I proceeded to look for a place to rent. I found a delightful house in the center of Dorset that was available in October.

Craig and I discussed my desire to be in Vermont and he was so supportive. He knew that I needed my girlfriends around me and that I felt alone in Chapel Hill. I decided to go for it. I held on to my bucket of

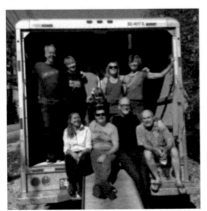

faith and asked the universe to take care of us, the delicate relationship of Cindy and Craig. I knew I would miss him terribly, but I also needed to take care of Cindy and put my oxygen mask on first. Craig, being a kind, loving, and caring soul, wanted to make sure I was not alone for the move and that I made it to Vermont in one piece, so he helped me move!

Off we went on a journey to Vermont driving a small U-Haul for twelve hours that was filled with what I needed to live. The drive was a great opportunity for us to catch up on life and to talk about "us." It was cathartic and healing, a step in the right direction that helped me feel at peace with the move. We were both welcomed with loving arms by several friends that helped us on "unloading" day!

That fall, I settled into my solo life in Vermont and continued running SHINE Strategy, which was truly blossoming with new brands like Vera Bradley and Orvis. Craig and I talked weekly and continued to share messages to keep each other laughing, but we also gave each other the space we needed. With each WhatsApp message, I still felt butterflies in my tummy with deep pangs of love. I couldn't ignore these pangs. I knew our souls were connected.

Carol, one of my closest friends, decided to host a "Bling on the Shine" party to celebrate my fiftieth birthday at the end of December. I discussed it with Craig and asked him to join the celebration and stay through New Year's Eve. The Bling on the Shine party was a huge success, and so was my visit with Craig. We had a great time as friends with benefits.

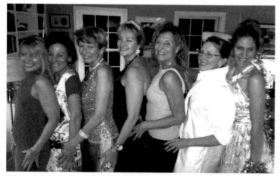

Me with Cindy, Carol, Lynn, Andrea, Terry, and Annette

On New Year's Day, we regrouped and had a serious conversation about our relationship. I was feeling so happy and in love that I didn't want Craig to go back to North Carolina. One of the things I love about Craig is his ability to take something complex and simplify it, which is what he did for us. He suggested we start "fresh" in the new year as if we were beginning to date again and building a new relationship. How romantic was that?! We planned monthly getaways organized by Craig. January, we met in New York City, February was North Carolina, and March was Boston. The monthly getaways were always romantic and full of adventures.

By the time April arrived, we both wanted to see each other more than once a month, so it became twice a month! By June, I opened my heart fully and was madly in love again with Craig. I loved his brilliance, sense of humor, caring spirit, unconditional love, and most of all our connection in mind, body, and spirit. Time helped me heal and strengthened my confidence in my new body, new business, and new life in Vermont. Yes, it was extremely hard going back and forth between Vermont and North Carolina, but we made it work. Eventually Craig moved to Vermont and then proposed to me on my fifty-fifth birthday!

We were planning a wedding for September 2020, but Covid happened, and we canceled. In 2019, we added Sunny, a yellow Lab puppy, to our family, who has been a tremendous source of love and joy for us. Instead of spending money on a wedding, we decided to buy a house together and combine our belongings. This has been one of the best things that has happened to us. Today, we are a very happy family with our life in Vermont. Great things do happen when we wait for them!

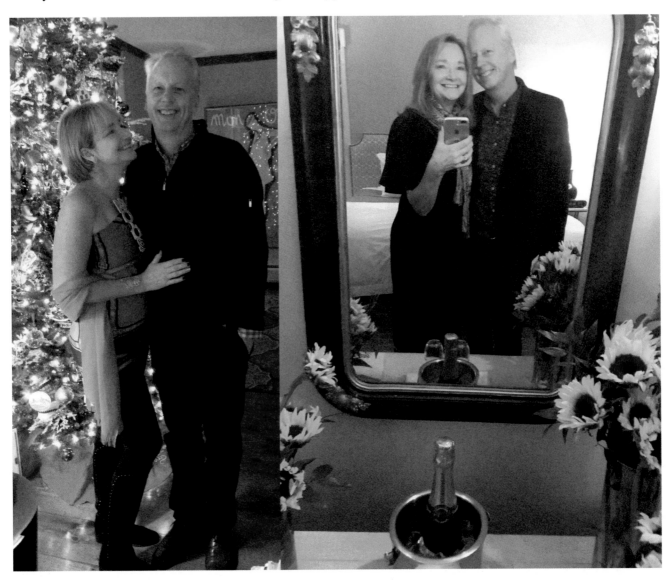

Why was I blessed to survive this? I have no idea, but what I do know is that I BELIEVED in me.

Chapter 26

LOOKING BACK ON
TEN YEARS . . .

It's hard for me to think that I am almost ten years cancer free. As I write this, I am one month away from the day I got my diagnosis. I still remember it like it was yesterday. It was one of the worst days of my life, yet I am here to tell my story, and many people can't say that because they didn't survive the journey. Why was I blessed to survive this? Was I chosen to spread my learnings, my strength, my mojo, and my belief in survival with others? I have no idea, but what I do know is that I BELIEVED in me, I BELIEVED in my doctors and nurses, I BELIEVED in my family and loved ones, and I BELIEVED that God had a purpose for me to carry on. I felt the light of the universe carry me through this tough journey of cancer, kind of like the poem, "Footprints in the Sand." God was and is always walking alongside me daily, experiencing the ups and downs of life's journey with me. From Joy and Delight to Grief and Sorrow (the main characters of the book *Cry, Heart, But Never Break* by Glenn Ringtved about death), I never felt let down. Yes, there were days I yelled and cried, "Why me?"; "I don't want to lose my hair!"; "I don't want to lose my breasts"; "I don't want to learn the new normal Cindy!"; and "I don't want to deal with hospitals, surgeries, medicine, recovery, sickness." I simply wanted life to stay as it was and remain happy.

I learned that happiness is a choice. We can choose each day to wake up happy and not sad or angry. To breathe and appreciate this gift of life. Yes, I still have bad days, but then I am reminded with each breath that the only thing we know for sure is that change is the nature of life. I am still here to experience change, so I let it go, breathe in and breathe out, knowing that everything is fine just the way it is. Be grateful to have your breath, to be present in this moment, to celebrate another birthday, to rejoice with love every day, and to cry when sad or emotional. Maybe this is the wisdom we are told we gain when we age, but age is just a number and we all have wisdom in our souls. You just need to listen to it, the voice inside your head that guides you.

I remember feeling like a failure because "I failed" at two marriages. All I ever dreamed of as a little girl was to be married, to be a loving wife, to play happy homemaker, to cook, to be a mother, caretaker, and nurturer. I tried marriage two times and I am grateful for these experiences. I was with my first husband for ten years and my second for fifteen years. We tend to repeat patterns, and I remember I tried to be something other than Cindy for each husband. I changed myself to be the "ski racer's wife" with my first husband because that is what I thought he wanted me to be. I changed myself to be the "professional sailor's wife" with my second husband. I was not a khakis and navy-blue blazer gal, but I thought I was supposed to be to make him happy. Bottom line, I changed myself to be what I thought others wanted, but at the end of the day, they wanted me, Cindy. Be yourself. This is your life and no one else's.

I think about my childhood and upbringing a lot. Was it the Barbie dolls I loved to play with that made me want to be a mother, housewife, and homemaker? No, it was the role models of my mother, my aunts, and my grandmothers that gave me this yearning. I wanted to be them and to do what they did. I came from an amazing, brilliant, and loving family! I am so proud and grateful to be part of this spectacular family lineage and to have learned from their life adventures and experiences. I learned how to deal with life's ups and downs together as an extended family unit. Most importantly, I learned about the importance of love, laughter, confidence, and belief.

- *LOVE is just a word until someone gives it meaning. My family taught me about being respectful to others and treating them how you wanted to be treated. My mother would also say, "Do unto others as you would have them do unto you!" My parents taught me about loving unconditionally with affection—holding hands, hugging, and kissing all the time. They were married sixty years. God bless them!*

- *LAUGHTER is what keeps us happy and young. There is nothing better than giggling with my life partner about something we did that was silly, having tickling matches with my brothers, squirming with laughter when my dad would blow bubbles on my belly, girlfriends giggling so hard we pee in our pants, and seeing your team members, friends, and family giggle with delight to see you! Shift life moments from mundane to memorable with humor and laughter.*

- *CONFIDENCE is the ability to believe in yourself, your superpowers, your intuition, and your innate knowledge. We all have confidence because we are born with it. Not all of us were fortunate enough to have parents that pat you on the back and tell you how great you are and what a fabulous job you did. Confidence can be hidden inside of us, but we need to learn how to use it, how to build up our own self-esteem, and how to take care of ourselves first. As a leader in business, it can be lonely at the top. You must learn to have confidence or you fail. If you believe in yourself, your confidence will shine through. As they say on airplanes, put your face mask on first before assisting others.*

- *BELIEF is about always carrying your "bucket of faith" with you, believing in yourself and your ability to tackle whatever crap comes your way, even a life-threatening disease. This belief allowed me to "Get On It and Kick Cancer's Butt"—at least my cancer. We have a long way to go to cure cancer for all. I believe in my angels above, the heavenly spirit, the universe of souls, and myself to carry on. This faith allowed me to not be afraid of dying. Releasing this fear allowed me to release the fear of losing a job (which I lost during chemo), the fear of my unknown future, and the fear of life without breasts. Because I believed in me and life, I wasn't afraid of what would happen next, and I let life happen. You've got to believe; without hope, fear and anger will dominate.*

My biggest lesson from this ten-year journey is to put my oxygen mask on first and to take care of myself before assisting others. I had been taking care of others for forty-eight years, and breast cancer taught me it was time to take care of Cindy. Don't let that happen to you! We only have one life to live and it's a gift! Every day you should wake up grateful to be alive and to experience each new breath. I do! Breathe in love; breathe out peace. Breathe in gratitude; breathe out love. Breathe in joy; breathe out happiness. Breathe in belief; breathe out confidence. Breathe in sunshine; breathe out light.

Someone once told me we can't have it all. Well, they are wrong. We CAN have it all, just not all at the same time. I had my breasts with sensitive nipples for forty-eight years. I know what it's like to feel their sensation and pleasure. I gave them up to save my life, and that's OK.

I had long healthy hair and a vibrant young body. Hair grows and the human body is resilient; they both bounce back as long we love and care for them.

My hope is that my story will help you take away a new meaning of positivity and gain confidence, strength, and inspiration to deal with your daily journey of life! Breathe ON! SHINE ON!

A Love Note to My Body:

First, I want to say thank you. Thank you for the heart you keep beating even when it's broken. Thank you for every answer you gave me in my gut. Thank you for loving me back when I didn't know to love you. Thank you for every time you recovered when I pushed you past our limits. Thank you for TODAY and for WAKING UP.

Thank you for every time you recovered when I pushed you past our limits. Thank you for TODAY and for WAKING UP!

Cindy is one of the
most courageous people
I have ever met.

Chapter 27

YOUR MASTER CLASS IN LIFE

By Laura Ravo

From the first time I met Cindy, I knew she was a force of nature. I was new to my role, joining a company in the middle of a pandemic. My business was in trouble in every sense of the word, and I needed help—fast. I made a few calls to the fearless leaders in Women in Retail Leadership and there she was, my dame in shining armor. One chat with her, and she jumped into action. Within twenty-four hours, she assessed the situation. Within forty-eight hours, we had a plan. Within seventy-two hours, she had called in reinforcements. And the rest was history—we lived to fight another day.

Her life lessons are woven into the tapestry of this book and are one woman's lessons in courage, tenacity, love, and fragility. Grab a pen or pencil and some paper. This is your master class in life.

Courage

What woman doesn't want to be courageous? It's something we all aspire to be, but how many of us actually would describe ourselves as courageous? It is a trait generally reserved for those who take extraordinary risks and/or superheroes. I beg to differ.

Cindy is one of the most courageous people I have ever met. She has the superhero cape to prove it. She can do absolutely anything she sets her mind to. Her ability to navigate the fear of her treatment through a simple decision tree exercise teaches us that fear is fear itself. A situation that seems daunting on the surface can be reframed into choices and possible outcomes, allowing us to shift from fear and anger to reason and peace.

Her bucket of faith and her unwavering belief in the power of prayer are lessons in surrender. There is power in acknowledging the fact that we are all exactly where we should be at any given moment and that mountains, no matter how high, are only temporary obstacles.

Tenacity

In its most basic form, it is determination, persistence; some even call it guts or grit. It is our ability to muscle through life and continue to move forward, despite the odds.

Cindy's mental strength and conviction are evident in her treatment journey and are rooted in her belief in her friends, her family, her angels, her faith, and most importantly herself. She busts the myth that we have to do it alone by showing us the power of a clearly defined support system that holds us up every step of the way.

Most importantly, Cindy reminds us that we are enough. During the many phases of her diagnosis, and after getting fired, she had some deep soul searching to do. Her confidence was shattered. She was battling cancer full on, and she vowed to "Get on it!" She teaches us that instead of giving up, the key is to double down on what is really important in life—including starting your own business. Her self-realization is an important reminder the answers have been in us all along. In the words of Maya Angelou, "You alone are enough. You have nothing to prove to anybody."

Love

Love is hard, really hard. Love is vulnerable. Love is risky. Love is everything! Cindy shows us YOU choose the way YOU want to live your life. Doing the hard work of self-discovery after two marriages, she finds the courage, strength, and vulnerability to let Craig all the way into her life and her heart.

She teaches us that love ALWAYS wins. The deep friendships she has built with the Whoville tribe are based in love, mutual respect, admiration, and affection. That bond is simply unbreakable and becomes her support system that carries her through her darkest hours and shines bright with her in her finest times.

Fragility

Human life is fragile. In the blink of an eye, our lives can change forever. We have the tendency to live our lives with the illusion of permanence, but it is just that, an illusion.

Cindy was on top of her game until her world was turned upside down after finding a lump. Nothing was ever the same—ever. She was never the same. Her journey teaches us that time is not a renewable resource and that we should not waste a moment of living. She vows to live each day to the fullest and if you know her, this is EXACTLY who she is. Cindy teaches us that saying yes to life is way more powerful than saying no. Tomorrow is just not guaranteed.

Cindy teaches us that saying yes to life is way more powerful than saying no. Tomorrow is just not guaranteed.

THANK YOU to everyone who supported me along my journey and shared your love with me! You know who you are!

ACKNOWLEDGMENT AND GRATITUDE

Writing a book is harder than I thought and more rewarding than I could have ever imagined. None of this would have been possible without my best friend, lover, fiancé, and hot male nurse, Craig Waller. Craig supported me through every low and celebrated the highs in style. He cared for and loved me unconditionally when I was sick, always putting me first. And he never gave up on me, even when I moved to Vermont and while I wrote this book!

To my incredible Chapel Hill medical team at UNC Lineberger Comprehensive Cancer Center for saving my life and making me feel like I was your only patient, thank you. I am grateful for the love, care, and medical attention you gave me, and for awarding me my Tar Heel pin!

I'm eternally grateful for my caregivers and support team of Mary, Fran, Vicky, Sarah, Linh, Tom, Zully, Barb, JD, Andrea, Terry, and Mary and Ed Norton. They helped me with doctor's appointments, airport runs, providing meals, grocery shopping, moral support, bathing me, shaving my legs, and cleaning my house! I could not have done this without you all.

Writing a book about the story of my breast cancer journey was a surreal process. I'm forever indebted to Paula Black, my professional coach and book publisher. She was instrumental in helping me make time to write, holding me accountable, managing the production, leading the design and editing process, and teaching me how to tighten my story.

I am extremely grateful for the recent gift of Laura Ravo in my life. She provided editorial help, keen insight, and ongoing support in bringing my stories to life. Laura helped me simplify my key lessons into four words: courage, tenacity, love, and fragility, and she summarized them into a master class!

To my family, friends, and business colleagues who supported me during my breast cancer treatment and surgeries, my shoulder and hand surgery, and my new life in Vermont, your fountain of love was overflowing, and you went out of your way to spoil me with gifts, cards, food, and humor!

Finally, I want to recognize the people that were part of my tribe and support team but have since passed on to the heavens: Mom and Dad Cozier, Clark, Nancy and Christie Whitcomb, Stu Jones, Dr. Amos, Shawn McKenna, Liz Cook, Andrea Diehl, Lynn Achee, Michael Munson, Brian Cabral, Kim and Tim Woodhouse, Jennifer Scarbrough, Mary Batchelor, Vince Lijoi, Jaguar, and Poppy.

Made in the USA
Columbia, SC
01 April 2022